Dr Arati Bhatia has spent forty years in diagnostics pathology, twenty-two of them as a professor at the University College of Medical Sciences, Delhi University. She obtained her MBBS from Amritsar Medical College in 1971 and a MD Pathology from AIIMS in 1976. She has also seen the medical profession from the other side as a caregiver and a cancer survivor.

CANCER, YOUR BODY AND YOUR DIET

A Vital Journey

Dr Arati Bhatia

SPEAKING TIGER

SPEAKING TIGER PUBLISHING PVT. LTD
4381/4, Ansari Road, Daryaganj
New Delhi 110002

First published in paperback by Speaking Tiger 2018

ISBN: 978-93-88326-11-7
eISBN: 978-93-88326-14-8

10 9 8 7 6 5 4 3 2 1

Typeset in Sabon Roman by SÜRYA, New Delhi
Printed at Gopsons Papers Ltd.

In memory of Arun Chacko,
and others who fought on bravely.

He has achieved success who has lived well, laughed often, and loved much;
Who has enjoyed the trust of pure women, the respect of intelligent men and the love of little children;
Who has filled his niche and accomplished his task;
Who has never lacked appreciation of Earth's beauty or failed to express it;
Who has left the world better than he found it,
Whether an improved poppy, a perfect poem, or a rescued soul;
Who has always looked for the best in others and given them the best he had;
Whose life was an inspiration;
Whose memory a benediction.

—Bessie Anderson Stanley

Contents

Health Tips for Preventing and Living with Cancer

Introduction

There is hope as long as there is life.

I write this from an unusual vantage point. First, from the perspective of an academician—being a pathologist, I studied, taught and diagnosed cancer for forty years, and have the knowledge to comprehend the changes in the body which give rise to cancer. Second, I was diagnosed with cancer in December 2008 and received the conventional treatment that was recommended at the time, including surgery, chemotherapy and radiation; thus I write from first-hand experience of the disease. Third, I write from the point of view of a counsellor—to the many patients I diagnosed, and to the friends who came seeking help because of my medical background. Finally, I have the viewpoint of a caregiver—my husband was diagnosed with stage IV prostate cancer in May 2010; his disease was already in the bones, the prognosis was grave, and chemotherapy of one kind or the other was the only treatment on offer.

I realized, over the duration of my husband's treatment, how much it helped him when I explained in simple terms how the cancer had developed and the ways in which it could behave in response to treatment. He was able to understand and actively participate in treatment decisions, and anticipate how these therapies could potentially benefit him.

When confronted with cancer, irrespective of the treatment strategy, and whatever the stage of the disease, food is possibly one of the most important uplifting factors. Advice on diet, however, from members of the attending medical team, is often sketchy at best. Most patients have numerous questions: What dietary precautions could be taken before starting treatment which would ease the side-effects? What changes in the diet would help with adequate food intake in the first few days post-chemotherapy? What modifications in the diet could help maintain a stable body weight so that a constant dosage of the drug could continue to be administered?

We needed answers taking into consideration my husband's eating habits and tastes, and also including all the ingredients for maintaining normal body function, for providing energy, for tissue repair during and after treatment, and for the removal of toxic waste. Finding no satisfactory solution to all these queries in any one place, I spent months researching and experimenting with diet for my husband, and found the exercise rewarding—a clear improvement in his quality of life.

My experience convinced me of the need for simplified information in the public domain so that people—patients, caregivers and healthcare-providers—can be empowered with the necessary insights into the day-to-day aspects of living with cancer. In the first part of this book, I have covered many aspects of the disease—its diagnosis, why it occurs, the impact and outcome of the diagnosis on the patient and the family. The second part focuses on the relationship between cancer and diet in the Indian context. Here, I discuss what foods should be avoided; what kind of diet can help in cancer prevention; and what essential nourishment should be provided during treatment (chemotherapy, surgery and radiotherapy), and during palliative care. I also suggest daily schedules for ailing patients, during and post-treatment, along with solutions to other common difficulties faced by cancer patients, after diagnosis and during treatment. The last section is an account of my personal experiences with my husband's battle against cancer; I hope that readers will find reading about such a candid history helpful in their own experience.

Dr Arati Bhatia

New Delhi

October 2018

Part I

WHAT IS CANCER?

Facts About Cancer

Diseases cannot be reduced to pathological facts, they constitute other worlds.

—Oliver Sacks

Historically, the Ramayana records the earliest evidence of treatment for a malignant tumour by the knife and by arsenical compounds.[1] In today's terms, this would be described as surgery and chemotherapy, respectively. Hippocrates (375-460 BCE) coined the word *karkinoma* derived from the Greek word *karkinos*, meaning crab.[2] Subsequently, this name stuck because of medicine's inability to get rid of malignant tumours and their capacity to infiltrate and attach themselves to adjacent tissue. In eras gone by, reports of cancer were anecdotal at best—not like the escalated rampant disease that we witness today, where almost every family knows of someone afflicted by cancer. What went wrong?

We live longer, for one. The sea of carcinogens or cancer-causing substances surrounding us—be it in the food we eat, the water we drink, or in the environment—has that much more time to work on our bodies. Most of these carcinogens, which have also increased exponentially over time, are our own, human creations. In our daily swim, we manage to navigate through most of them without serious impact. This is due to inherent factors, namely a healthy body and a sound mind. In fact, despite these trying circumstances, we have an infinite ability to heal ourselves.

The development of cancer in our body is a multi-step process and is slow to unfold. How long a cancer really takes to develop is difficult to predict. It could be months or years. To begin with, these changes can be easily corrected by our own defence mechanisms, primarily through the immune system and the 'molecular policeman' of the cell—the p53 gene. The immunological and biological surveillance that exists in our body manages to remove mutated or abnormal cells—as in the case of infectious organisms—and we continue to live in a state of good health.

It is believed that the DNA mutations (alteration in the chemical structure of DNA) that lead to the development of cancer occur on several occasions during our lifetime. Mostly, the body comes out healthy, having eliminated the mutation. At other times, the mutations progress further in a multi-step process, and eventually evolve into cancer over a period of time. The factors responsible for the switching 'on' of the cancer trigger are not exactly known, but poor general health, improper nutrition, environmental factors and stress are a few suspects in the long list of probabilities.

Although tumours may appear at any age, they are most likely to occur in older individuals, suggesting that environmental factors may be at work. Another peak for malignant tumours is during childhood, but this is quite distinct from the adult form of the disease, as it arises in organs or tissues with rapid growth, like bone marrow, bones and neural tissues. Rapidly growing tissue may be subject to mutations resulting in the development of cancer.

In their abnormal mutated state, the cancer cells manage to mask themselves and escape the fury of the immune system—they are immortalized and continue to grow unhindered, not responding to the signals from adjacent cells to stop multiplication. Moreover, they manage to requisition the surrounding normal tissues and their functions for their own growth and proliferation—at the expense of the host, just like a parasite.

Malignant tumours comprise rapidly multiplying cells that may be metabolically three times more active than normal tissues. Thus, the tumours sift out a greater portion of the nutrients present in blood circulation, that have been absorbed from food, for their own nutritional needs. This greatly reduces the availability of essential nutrients for the normal metabolic functions of the host cells—effectively starving them. Some cancer patients succumb directly to their tumours; more succumb indirectly, because of severe malnutrition. In this weakened condition the patient often develops an immune-deficient state and becomes highly susceptible to infections like pneumonia. Doctors and care-givers have consistently confronted a major challenge in cancer patients: reduced appetite, exacerbated by the treatments given—chemotherapy and/or radiation therapy. It is crucial therefore to provide a higher caloric diet to meet the additional nutrient needs of the patient, and to ensure that even if the patient can't eat very much, what they do eat is significantly nutritious.

Cancer is a complex disease characterized by multiple genetic and molecular alterations of the cells. These alterations involve fundamental changes in the ability of the body to: kill and dispose of old and abnormal cells; regulate unfettered multiplication of abnormal cells; control the abnormal cells' ability to break their moorings and locally infiltrate and destroy adjacent normal tissue; and/or their spread into distant organs. Therefore, surgical removal of tumours should include adequate excision of surrounding tissue, failing which local recurrence of the tumour is inevitable. Further, the tumour cells influence the growth of new blood vessels that carry nutrition to the developing cancer cells. For all these changes, the growing cancer depends entirely on the host for its nourishment. It then seems logical for us to look at our diet and introduce changes in our food habits that could interfere with tumour growth and keep cancer growth on hold.

We are aware of many substances whose abuse may cause cancer. Some of these, like tobacco, whether chewing or smoking, excessive consumption of alcohol, and aflatoxin in peanuts, can clearly be avoided. There are many carcinogenic substances however, which are invisible and therefore may be considered unavoidable. We are unaware of their presence in our food, our water, or in the environment, and even of their harmful effects. We need to work around these toxins: firstly by educating ourselves on the content of our diets, be it our food or what we drink; secondly, by introducing foods that may have a protective effect against cancer. Making a few changes in our food habits could go a long way in improving the state of our health.

One study suggested that only 5 to 10 per cent of cancers were attributable to genetic or intrinsic factors; 90 to 95 per cent of cancers have their roots in environmental toxins, infections and our lifestyle (i.e. extrinsic or epigenetic factors).[3] Cancer risk, therefore, is heavily influenced by extrinsic factors and only marginally by intrinsic ones. Further, a study conducted in the US revealed that 30 to 35 per cent of cancers were linked to diet, 25 to 30 per cent of cancer-related deaths were due to tobacco, while 15 to 20 per cent were due to infection.[4] Other minor causes were radiation, stress, lack of physical activity and pollution. The authors of this study suggest that cancer was a preventable disease that requires major lifestyle changes.

In the US, there has been a 25 per cent decline in cancer deaths over the last two decades. More than half can be attributed to cancer prevention strategies. The single most preventable cause of cancer is cigarette smoking. Decrease in tobacco use is largely responsible for this reduction—applying this logic to other known causes of cancers and avoiding them would result in the reduction of these preventable cancers.

Epigenetic factors are external or environmental factors that cause changes in the functioning and/or regulation of DNA without altering their primary sequence. These are factors that switch the genes ‘on’ and ‘off’, and affect how cells read the genes, or how the genes express themselves. Essentially, it is anything other than the DNA sequence or code that influences the development of the cell. Some common epigenetic factors that influence the development of cancer include deficiency of folic acid, smoking, heavy metals and pesticides, to name but a few. It is therefore believed that you can shift your gene expression through nutrition and lifestyle choices.

Is psychological stress the cause or an effect of cancer? Though stress has no direct link in the causation of cancer, repeatedly dealing with stressful situations over long periods of time can cause health problems. The body responds to stress by releasing stress hormones (epinephrines) that not only increase the blood pressure and heart rate but raise the blood sugar levels, which may be responsible for a weakened immune system.

Stress may result in behavioural changes; for instance, increased smoking in smokers, overeating and obesity, or an increased intake of alcohol. All these changes increase cancer risk and, in fact, are extremely unhealthy choices. On the other hand, a diagnosis of cancer definitely causes stress, from the time of diagnosis all through treatment and even after its completion. The stress of whether there will be tumour recurrence never truly goes away.

The Diagnosis of Cancer

The truth is not for all men, but only for those who seek it.

—Ayn Rand

It is said that cancer creeps in slowly and therefore, it is often referred to as a 'silent killer'. There are more than 300 types of malignancies that may involve the many organs of the body. If the cancer occurs on the skin, like a non-healing ulcer or an inflamed mole, it is likely to draw attention and can be detected earlier because of its visibility. The important point is not to ignore any lumps in the head, neck, breast or elsewhere, or ulcers in the mouth or tongue that persist, even though they may not produce significant symptoms. It is the cancers that lie in deep organs that go undetected, and often spread beyond the confines of the organ of origin by the time of diagnosis. Cancers of the pancreas or the ovary are examples of problematic, deep-seated malignancies that are largely diagnosed late.

Cancer may be diagnosed as part of routine annual examinations done to exclude malignancy or other ailments like heart disease, hypertension or diabetes, or when a person shows specific symptoms and weight loss to a healthcare professional. Only seldom do patients with cancer show up as medical emergencies with bleeding or intestinal obstruction. A diagnosis of cancer at an early stage in the disease is associated with good prognosis and survival.

A diagnosis of cancer does not have to spell doom. Early stage tumours have excellent prognosis. There is a huge variation in survival depending on the cancer type, organ involved, and the grade and stage of the disease. The method used to quantify the extent of disease, both locally and its spread in every patient, is designated as the 'stage' of the disease. The grade of a tumour is the level of differentiation or how closely the tumour resembles normal tissue. High grade tumours have poorer resemblance to the normal tissue and therefore poorer prognosis. However, survival rates have more than doubled in the last forty years. Improved survival is attributable to medical science and the development of early detection tools as well as the advancement of treatment modalities.

During cancer screening, routine blood and urine tests measure specific markers associated with some common cancers; when detected, the abnormality points the doctor towards the organ involved. Further investigations such as imaging procedures—computed tomography (CT) scans, ultrasounds, magnetic resonance imaging (MRIs), radionuclide bone scans, positron emission tomography (PET) scans—and/or biopsies are used to confirm the diagnosis and determine the extent of disease.

Over the years, as cancer treatment modalities depend entirely on an accurate, specific and comprehensive diagnosis, the laboratory diagnosis of cancer has evolved into a fine art. This tissue diagnosis is a prerequisite before treatment is started. Several diagnostic approaches are available: For instance, exfoliative cytology, or the study of cells shed from a tumour, is used in the female genital system (PAP smear). Sputum, urine, body fluids and cerebro-spinal fluid (CSF) are used to make a diagnosis of cancer through the examination of cytology smears. Fine needle aspiration cytology for tumours is a minimally invasive procedure and can be done in the lymph nodes, breasts, salivary glands, thyroid, lung and liver. Incision biopsy or excision of the tumour gives a final histological report. Frozen section examination is used to make a quick diagnosis, as well as to assess the margin for any residual tumour at the time of surgery. Sophisticated techniques like flow cytometry and molecular markers are used to further categorize some tumours. Many tumour markers are used to diagnose and follow up with the cancer patient.

Once the diagnosis of cancer is established by pathology and/or radiology, it is then 'staged' to determine its extent. Baseline blood investigations are done for further monitoring. Only after these are completed are the available treatment options—in accordance with standard protocols—offered to the patient. Then the treatment time frame is worked out and the treatment is started.

The type of treatment given depends on the pathology of the cancer cells and the stage. Out of surgery, chemotherapy and radiation therapy, any one, or a combination of two or more regimens can be selected. The importance of the accuracy of the pathology opinion cannot be overstated. It is based on this report after all that the treatment is given!

It is an all-out war once the treatment starts. If the cancer is likened to a terrorist outfit, a multi-pronged attack against it is justifiable. To achieve this, the terrorist and its accomplices must be found and eliminated (surgery/radiation therapy); their support system of funding and communication must also be destroyed, and sleeper cells must be identified and taken out (chemotherapy). Only then will there be complete annihilation of the cancer.

In some tumours, like breast and lung cancer, additional tests on the tumour tissue are necessary to determine the complete nature of the cancer before embarking on the treatment. Knowing all the potential targets in a tumour and selecting drugs to strike them all provides the greatest likelihood of effective elimination of all cancer cells, thereby achieving complete remission. A couple of years after my husband Arun's diagnosis, a friend faced a dilemma. She had undergone surgery after a diagnosis of breast cancer. It was oestrogen (ER) and progesterone (PR) receptor positive but the HER2 (human epithelial growth factor receptor 2) was equivocal. Being positive for HER2 would offer her an additional tool against the cancer cells (see p. 35 in 'Targeted Therapy'). My advice to her at the time was to get a second opinion on the slides with a repeat of the markers—HER2 in particular—by fluorescence in-situ hybridization (FISH), a more sensitive test for the detection of HER2 than the routine test done in most laboratories.[5] She got her slides reviewed, and the HER2 turned out to be positive when FISH was used, giving her an additional drug for specifically targeting her tumour cells.

In another instance, a seventy-five-year-old golfer developed slowly increasing symptoms pertaining to prostate enlargement—not uncommon at his age. His golfing partner suggested a visit to the urologist. The blood and urine examination did not reveal anything untoward. A prostate biopsy was diagnosed as high-grade cancer, and treatment was started. His condition progressively deteriorated and he slowly developed renal failure three months later.

His nephew, a doctor, visited him and asked for a review of the biopsy slides. Two days later, the review returned a diagnosis of high-grade bladder cancer. This explained the almost normal levels of prostate-specific antigen (PSA), a substance produced by the prostate gland at the time of diagnosis and the complete lack of response to treatment directed against prostate cancer. The renal failure was due to the obstruction caused in the ureter, i.e. the tube that drains the urine from the kidney to the urinary bladder. The original erroneous biopsy report was the result of the infiltration of the bladder tumour into the prostate. A second opinion before the start of treatment could have averted inappropriate therapy, waste of money and loss of time.

The Importance of Communication

To my friend with the HER2 positive breast cancer, I had suggested that she interview a couple of oncologists before starting her treatment, and choose one that she was most comfortable with. Someone who communicated well, was not in a hurry, did not bark orders and was willing to explain each situation to her when it was required.

It is our ability to communicate—not just the raw emotions of fear, happiness and anger, but our abilities to vocalize the details of our daily experiences—that sets us apart from the animal kingdom. It is strange, then, that communication skills are not actively emphasized during medical education. And many doctors, as a result, are poor communicators.

The only emphasis in medical education is on excellence in subject knowledge and in associated medical or surgical skills. The most important human aspect of medicine—the ability to communicate with the patient—gets little priority, under the assumption that this skill will develop naturally with practice. This clearly does not happen in many cases—patients need doctors to listen, and then list treatment options, weigh the pros and cons of each alternative with the patient, and help them make informed decisions.

Getting greater clarity on the disease and treatment process benefits the patient emotionally and reduces suffering. It also improves participation and commitment to treatment, even though it may have little impact on the outcome. I recall the case of Dr B who went to England to get his Fellowship of the Royal College of Surgeons (FRCS). He was outstanding as far as knowledge and skills were concerned, but he was rejected for the job and asked to return six months later after improving his communication skills. Upon achieving this, he was told the job was his for the asking. Automatic mastery in communication comes naturally only to a few doctors—most have only learnt by emulating their teachers and observing others.

This acquired skill of good communication that builds trust does wonders for patient compliance in various diseases, including cancer. The doctor must place all necessary facts related to the disease and its treatment before the patient before embarking on the medication. Doctors in India are highly qualified and skilled in their specialties, but they often fail in their ability to communicate. They sometimes reduce their interactions to making mere pronouncements. Some patients have education and access to the internet, and require expert information to gain understanding of their disease in order to make it easier to cope with the consequences. The less educated deserve no less of an explanation, and a discussion about the treatment options—especially for a disease like cancer, where the entire family is heavily invested in the patient's well-being and the financial implications are huge.

The Internet

The internet is a useful tool for finding information on cancer, and for connecting with other patients and caregivers. However, there is controversy among the medical fraternity regarding patients reading about their cancers online. Some feel that this should be avoided as patients may interpret the information erroneously, which could be counter-productive and add to their anxiety. This view may be particularly true about reading survival statistics, which are both confusing and frightening. Others feel that reading empowers the patient and the wealth of information is reassuring, allowing them better control over their decision-making.

It is difficult to ascertain the reliability of the medical information, since the internet is not regulated. Good judgement while searching for internet data becomes critical. When in doubt, run the information past the healthcare team for clarity. There may be wisdom in getting the doctor's recommendation on websites for reliability. This would ensure accuracy and credibility of the source.

Another issue that needs consideration is the fact that medical science is constantly evolving. As newer remedies gain the US Food and Drug Administration's (FDA) approval and come into the market, the internet gets bombarded with information on these newer options. This data can be accessed by the patient or caregiver, who then becomes aware of these newer drugs and their utility in their cancer. Since the internet is ubiquitous in many Indian households, doctors should be open to the idea of discussing information gleaned from the internet if the patient brings it up.

Caregivers frequently join care groups to keep abreast of the situation they find themselves in. A neighbour of ours was diagnosed with chronic lymphocytic leukaemia (CLL) at an age when this disease was still considered uncommon—she was only forty-one then. She had repeated relapses and many types of infections, including fungal pneumonia because of low immunity, but her spirit never failed her. She even developed lymphoma of the ovary and lost an eye. Finally, a bone-marrow transplant cured her. Years later, I asked how she managed to smile through everything. She said, 'I didn't want to know the negative outcomes of the disease—it was my husband who joined the CLL group online and had discussions with the other patients. I never corresponded, but he kept me updated with all the positive feedback.' She had found the perfect solution for herself for maintaining a positive frame of mind. She understood that knowledge about other people's complications would have impacted her negatively. Her husband on the other hand, the caregiver, was prepared for every eventuality.

Grappling with the Diagnosis

The oldest and strongest emotion of mankind is fear. The oldest and strongest kind of fear is fear of the unknown.

—H.P. Lovecraft

A diagnosis of cancer brings our worst fears to the forefront. For some, it is almost like an end-of-life experience. The initial reaction to a cancer diagnosis can be devastating, and it is probably one of the most trying times in the entire cancer experience. The turmoil, the feelings that race through the mind, often leave one utterly unsure of oneself, or of one's ability to deal with the situation. There is confusion, uncertainty, anger, fear, betrayal and frustration—all at the same time. Sometimes, a sense of denial leaves one in utter disarray. One may also question the body's ability to put up even a token resistance against the disease. These emotions become so overwhelming that it is difficult to see any light at the end of the tunnel. Within a moment, life changes forever. As one cancer patient described it, 'It brought me to my knees.'

These reactions and emotions are normal, even as the task ahead is daunting. There are many imponderables, including the impact of this diagnosis on the family. Coping with the treatment or even losing a body part is difficult to comprehend to begin with, but discussing your worries with the doctor, the caregiver (family members like parents, spouse, brother, sister, son, daughter or even a friend), and with members of the support group, even a priest, helps calm the mind and bring the disease into perspective. Whatever helps to acquire a positive frame of mind should be attempted to tide over these testing times. Cancer patients with a strong support group survive longer.[6]

A good doctor-patient relationship is central to dealing with and overcoming the initial hardships, and it ultimately determines treatment success. However, this is only one part of it. A positive relationship helps develop trust, encourages greater patient participation and confidence in the treatment. Moreover, the caregiver also benefits, since discussion about the cancer, potential treatment modalities, and likely outcomes gives him or her a holistic view which improves understanding. Later, as treatment continues, acceptance of the diagnosis sinks in, which finally helps the patient cope better with their ordeal.

In India, the interaction is usually limited to only the oncologist and the patient. In most hospital setups, a counsellor, a dietician, and support group members are missing from the discussion. The treatment offered in cancer hospitals is for the disease alone and not for the patient as a whole. Other health professionals, apart from the oncologist, should also be involved since supportive care from them will help patients live a more complete life despite the cancer. The eventual goal is to cure or control the cancer; however, until such a state is reached, there will be a need to relieve pain or other symptoms, maintain general health and nutrition, and improve the quality of life by providing emotional, psychological and logistical support to the patient. Additionally, a holistic discussion gives clarity to the caregiver. No one addresses, at the time of diagnosis, the problems that may arise during treatment or when it fails. Family and friends become caregivers, but they often suffer from extreme anxiety and completely lack any guidance. Who will provide support to the caregiver?

Strategies for Coping

For some, spiritual guidance may be at the core of treatment success. The true essence of this guidance lies in its ability to invoke mental strength, which enhances peace of mind.

Prayers have been found to relieve stress, and create a sense of meaning, purpose and solace. Individuals who are spiritually inclined may have greater benefit and suffer less anxiety and depression, finding strength to cope with their disease.

Meditation is also useful. It alleviates anxiety and helps in pain management. One of the simplest methods of meditation is single-point concentration where we choose an object and then meditate solely on it. It promotes relaxation, builds internal strength, and helps develop compassion, love and forgiveness. Single-pointedness can be achieved by using beads or repeating mantras. It is often used to clear the mind, and ease health concerns by lowering the blood pressure, and reducing depression and anxiety.

Though Arun's visits to the church were limited to four or five per year, he was a firm believer in religion and a member of the Cathedral Church of the Redemption. The Sunday after his diagnosis, he came back after attending an hour-long service. He was at peace with himself—after his initial silence and negative attitude, stemming from his dislike for hospitals and fear of needles. He was calmer, all his doubts were gone and he was willing to undergo treatment. He quickly overcame these phobias and learned to cope with his disease mainly through discussion. It is all about how an event is perceived—is it seen as traumatic or is there a perception that it can be dealt with? Resilience is a skill that can be taught and individuals with spiritual and religious support are more likely to develop it. This resilience may prevent the adverse event from becoming traumatic.

A journalist friend who had also struggled with cancer wrote to me about his experience in dealing with the disease: 'Even though the news shattered me, my exposure to Buddhist teachings helped me to cope with the aftermath. Even now, I periodically sense the dread rising up in me, but instead of my mind barrelling down a spiral of depression and dread, it takes a pause and tries to soothe itself, by remembering the truth so beautifully taught by the Buddha. And the Buddhist perspective on life helps to see things in clearer light and the unstable, fearful mind gets some solace. It is an extremely internal journey, often ineffable.'

Religious beliefs work differently for different people. A technician brought his ten-year-old niece for some laboratory tests. The child had been very sick, pale, and unable to stand with extreme bone pain over the last twenty days. She was diagnosed as having acute leukaemia, and was advised chemotherapy. She came for the treatment with her father. Her mother had been immersed in prayers for the last two days. Five days after the therapy, it seemed like the malignancy had just melted away. She could not only stand but she was walking and was completely pain-free. The mother was convinced that this miracle was the answer to her prayers, and that her daughter was cured. The family returned to the village believing that prayers were the answer. Five months later, we were told that the little girl had passed away.

Sometimes people react towards the other extreme. A friend's father—a guardian of his faith who never wavered in reading the Guru Granth Sahib for over seventy years—was diagnosed with bladder cancer. He was completely shattered and unforgiving that, even after having lived his life in accordance with his Guru's teachings, he had developed cancer. Why was he being punished? Overnight, from being an ardent follower he lost his faith, feeling completely isolated and let down.

Importance of Nutrition

While the diagnosis is being established and treatment modalities are being determined, it is crucial to provide the patient a diet with all the nutrients, i.e. calories, proteins, vitamins and minerals, that support their health. Normal food quantities prior to illness should be maintained.

Recommended Diet Post-Diagnosis

Start the day with fresh fruit juice (see p. 97).

Breakfast:

Sugar-free cereal with flax seeds, walnuts and cinnamon OR eggs and toast OR upma with vegetables OR besan ke cheele
Coffee/tea.

Lunch:

Dal,
Vegetables (not including potatoes),
Salad,
Curd,
Roti/rice
Fruit.

Evening tea:

A cup of tea
1 unsweetened biscuit (optional).

Dinner (cooked either Indian or Western style):

One non-vegetarian or vegetarian dish (meat/fish/chicken/paneer/dal)
Vegetables
Salad,
Rice/roti.

Others:

Green/black tea thrice daily.
Wheatgrass juice once a day (see box on p. 100).
Avoid alcohol.

Quality of Life

The quality of life is more important than life itself.

—Alexis Carrel

Life, as a concept taught to a child, pertains to anything that can breathe, reproduce, grow, excrete, react to stimuli, and perhaps move. For all these activities, food is a fundamental requirement. Religion and philosophy would include social ties, consciousness, happiness, ethics and morality in their definitions of life. While the pursuit of well-being is a goal for all religion, philosophy and science, for a cancer patient, life is all about nutrition and maintaining quality of life.

According to the Oxford English Dictionary, quality of life is the 'standard of health, comfort, and happiness experienced by an individual or group.' One must note that it is defined in terms of health and happiness, and not wealth.

The World Health Organization (WHO) defines quality of life as 'an individual's perception of their position in life in the context of the culture and value systems in which they live and in relation to their goals, expectations, standards and concerns.'[7] The Wong Baker face scale that measures pain adds the concept of time to this definition, stressing that quality of life applies 'at a precise moment of time'.[8] In other words, quality of life can mean happiness, that is, the subjective state of the mind rather than the 'standard of living'.

A number of different conditions affect one's quality of life, including objective aspects like social, environmental and economic factors, as well as subjective perceptions dependent upon the individual's needs and priorities. These components vary from country to country and from urban to rural areas. The factors are individualistic and depend on what is the baseline or the happiness requirement specific for each person. Measuring the parameters of quality of life may be difficult, as it influences individuals differently. In some cases, a situation like the loss of a job or a setback in business may have a profound impact, while others may handle it better.

From the healthcare perspective, there are many variables affecting quality of life, but they are difficult to define clearly. The most common ones often include physical health, psychological state, and life satisfaction. The latter means that not just the absence of disease, but the presence of physical, mental and social well-being, fulfilment of personal expectations and acceptance of the existing situation—all are integral to quality of life. These may develop over time, permitting the patient to work towards making the best of a difficult situation. The realization that, even though many activities are restricted but the requirements for happiness are still achievable, is a huge boost to morale.

Subjective well-being depends upon one's perception at two separate points in time—with and without the disease. While the longevity of human life has increased due to advancement in medical science, our attention should always be focused on the quality of life. For the medical profession, quality of life has different connotations related to life and living. In any chronic illness, where the patient may eventually get incapacitated, the quality of life is an important index of their general well-being. The essential ingredients of quality of life are the standards of health, comfort and happiness. Basic medical care places considerable emphasis on the patient's ability to enjoy normal-life activities. Though, it is primarily dependent on the subjective evaluation of the positive and negative aspects of life in general, it is an essential concept in health. Some diseases and forms of treatments can impair the quality of life, but as long as the individuals achieve their personal goals, hopes and aspirations, it may be considered reasonable.

When it comes to cancer care and research, quality of life is an important consideration. Illness-related factors may affect the quality of life in cancer patients. Such patients experience a wide variety of symptoms and side-effects; inadequate management of these can hamper the patient's daily activities, while treatment can relieve suffering.[9] The symptoms may have varied results: subtle and inconsequential for some, while for others they may be pronounced. For cancer patients, the level of distress experienced by the individual directly affects their quality of life. In many cases, as in breast cancer treatment, questionnaires are routinely used to assess quality of life during treatment.[10]

Quality of life is now also being used as an outcome measure in studies to evaluate the effectiveness of treatments like chemotherapy when there is progression of the disease. It has become an important end point for treatment. It can even be said that poor quality of life is an early indicator of disease progression. Therefore, the treating doctor and caregivers need to have an understanding of how the disease affects an individual, and how to guide them through these situations. Taking into account the patient's quality of life improves the relationship between them and the patients, resulting in more comprehensive healthcare.

Why Did Cancer Develop?

We may never understand illnesses such as cancer. In fact, we may never cure it. But an ounce of prevention is worth more than a million pounds of cure.

—David Agus, author of *The End of Illness*

Why did cancer develop? This question needs answers. Why did only two people out of three in my family develop cancer? I must admit that we were both of the same age, just three months apart; but genetically totally different—one was of North Indian descent, the other a Maratha-Kerala combination. It was certainly not genetic—no one in either family had had similar cancers.

So what had gone wrong? What were the common factors we shared, besides age?

This discussion may be in the realm of speculation, but it needs scrutiny and awareness. Neither of us smoked, drank or was obese. So where had we transgressed? Was it the food we ate? Was it the environment we lived in? A combination of these factors? Or was it simply a coincidence?

The human body is made up of millions of cells with many different functions. Similar cells come together to form tissues, these tissues form organs, and different organs work together to form organ systems. There are many such organ systems that work in agreement with each other, in perfect equilibrium with the mind, to form a healthy functioning body. It is much like an orchestra, where different sounds from the various instruments blend together to produce the perfect euphony that is so uplifting. Somehow, this harmony can be lost and a disease like cancer can take root.

The Development of Cancer

Cancer is, possibly, the unfortunate by-product of evolution.

Our complicated structure makes us vulnerable to this disease. Human development begins from a single cell. Exponential cell divisions result in the formation of our complex anatomy. The formation of organ systems requires many signals, along with the natural trimming of unwanted cells by the process of 'cell death' or apoptosis, to arrive at the final product—a human.

It is a miracle how a single cell first becomes a mass of cells and then forms a hollow structure that will form all the organs of the body. Nine months later, a perfectly formed baby emerges with all its organs in place—all from that original, single cell. The organs may be the tube-like structures of the gastrointestinal system or the heart and blood vessels, or the diverse group of solid organs such as the liver, kidney, spleen or brain—each distinctly different in structure and function. The entire process is controlled by the many biological signals from the cells that operate like clockwork, controlling the size, shape and placement of the various developed organs of the body.

All these structures, once completely developed, require maintenance to deal with the regular wear and tear that occurs during life. The various bodily functions are maintained at a constant rate by a process of cell division that replaces non-functional or senescent cells by functional ones, as and when required. This process is complex. A pathway of signals 'switch on' the multiplication. During this 'switch on', for whatever reason, some cells may get corrupted during cell division, leading to the development of abnormal or mutated cells. These are autonomous cells—completely out of control, and not influenced by the 'switch off' signals from the surrounding normal cells. They continue to multiply even after all the necessary replacement has been completed.

It is the proliferation of these abnormal cells over a long period of time which leads to the development of cancer. Cancer cells are a law unto themselves. They have an unstoppable momentum, enabling them to multiply in an unrestrained manner. One of the genes that control accidental cell growth, p53, undergoes change in its genetic structure in many types of cancers.

The p53 gene is also known as the 'guardian of the genome' and is one of the most common targets for genetic alterations. A little over fifty percent of human cancers have a mutation of this gene. The p53, the 'molecular policeman' that prevents the proliferation of corrupted cells and regulates several hundred genes, either thwarts the cell cycle (see p. 32) or triggers cell death (by apoptosis).

Loss of the function of the p53 results in DNA damage that goes unrepaired, and mutations accumulate. Usually, the biological surveillance of our body protects us by destroying the corrupted cells and keeping us out of harm's way. Failure of this biological surveillance leaves a tiny number of wayward cells that continue to grow unchecked. When these damaged cells multiply repeatedly, they produce a clone of abnormal cells which may march towards cancer formation.

To begin with, the cancer cells in a given tumour are similarly mutated. However, over time, as the tumour continues to grow unchecked, more and more mutations take place as all controls are lost. The resultant tumour is not only larger, but it has cells which are genetically more diverse, making it difficult to target during treatment. This may also be a factor responsible for the development of drug resistance during treatment (see p. 38 in 'Drug Resistance').

The main concern which began this chapter was that two members of the same family had developed cancer in organs sensitive to hormones, suggesting that somehow extraneous hormone-like substances played a role. These extraneous hormone-like substances are called xenoestrogens and are widespread in the environment.

The Causes

Doctors treat the cancer but do little to determine why it occurred. What were the toxic chemicals present in our body at the time of diagnosis that may have been responsible? Xenoestrogens from pesticides affect us directly when we consume chemically-grown, non-organic fruits and vegetables, from farm animals fed contaminated foods, and from plastics used in packaging. These toxins were virtually non-existent before World War II. Now they seem to be everywhere.

Man-made chemicals are all around us—from pesticides to cosmetics to baby bottles to computers and cell phones. It is impossible to determine how many of us are contaminated by these bio-accumulative and toxic substances! During their manufacture and use, these chemicals are released into the environment and absorbed by animals and humans alike. Due to slow degradation (or no degradation at all), they accumulate in our bodies, particularly in the fat. They are 'endocrine disruptive' chemicals which interfere with hormone systems in animals and humans, causing cancer, reproductive problems and damage to the DNA.

This is a bit like the DDT story. Dichloro-diphenyl-trichloroethane or DDT is a chlorinated hydrocarbon that remains in the environment for an indefinite period of time, without loss of potency. It was a synthetic insecticide first manufactured in 1940, and widely used to combat malaria, typhus and other insect-borne human diseases, as well as pests in crops, livestock and homes. Compounds such as DDT have reportedly caused massive loss to bird life, adversely affecting reproduction in some species. We belong to the generation which was overtly exposed to this chemical. It was considered the wonder solution that controlled mosquitoes by regular, liberal sprays both outside and sometimes inside the house. It even briefly eliminated malaria from India in the late 1980s. At that time, no one was aware of its toxicity. However, a high concentration of this compound has been found in the tissues of individuals exposed to it. DDT breaks down slowly. Today, it is banned in many countries for being carcinogenic.

The rising incidence of cancer may be linked to many factors. In 2014, the WHO suggested three important causes: environmental pollution, pesticides and excessive consumption of refined and processed foods.[11] Overnight, it may not be possible to change the environment we live in, or remove the pesticides completely from our food chain. After all, the soil is contaminated by them. But we can control and modify our diet.

The extent of this contamination is far-reaching. Polar bears eat large fish and seals. These, in turn, eat smaller fish, which eat even smaller fish. When the smallest fish have been contaminated by pesticides, so have the polar bears, even though they never left their pristine environment. They are at the top of the food chain just as we are, and like us, they have also been hit by pesticides.

Till not so long ago, Kanpur, Faridabad and Varanasi were among the most polluted cities in the world, and the situation is worsening every winter.[12] Therefore, there is no doubt that the air we breathe is foul, full of sulphur dioxide, carbon monoxide, ozone, nitrogen dioxide, lead and particulate matter.

What about our water supply? Even our most sacred river, the Ganges, is nothing but an open drain. Its waters are contaminated by sewage, chemicals, heavy metals and pesticides. What percentage of these substances remain in the water we drink? Or in the water we use for irrigation—which further contaminates our crops? The answer remains unknown. There is no check on the chemicals contaminating the soil, which are used for the cultivation of crops.

Despite overexposure to many more carcinogens in our environment, the incidents of lung, colon, breast and kidney cancers are much lower in India than in the West. Something is clearly working for us. Is it the thousands of gods we have or is it the food we eat? Could something in our diet, something which we haven't given much thought to, be protecting us?

Cancer Treatments

The secret of the care of the patient is in caring for the patient.

—Dr Francis Peabody

Surgery

Surgery is one of the treatment options available to some patients with cancer. It involves the removal of the tumour and the surrounding tissue by operating surgically on the patient. Surgery can either be performed in cancer patients to make a tissue diagnosis of cancer, where a small portion of the tumour is removed, or a complete excision of the malignant tumour is done when the diagnosis is unequivocal. Tumour removal may be curative when small in size, but mostly, surgery is combined with other treatment modalities such as radiation and/or chemotherapy.

Conventional surgery involves making a large incision, mostly through the skin and muscle, but sometimes through the bone, to remove the tumour. Less invasive methods are more popular now. They are offered to patients because of the advancement in imaging techniques which provide a complete picture, including the extent of tumour prior to surgery, and are associated with earlier recovery. **Debulking surgery** is done to remove as much of the tumour as possible—without causing too much damage to the surrounding normal tissue—in patients where the surgeon is unable to remove the entire cancer. At times, when the tumour is extensive, chemotherapy or radiation is given prior to the surgery to shrink the lesion.

Palliative surgery is used to relieve side-effects caused by the growing cancer in cases that are otherwise inoperable due to the stage and extent of local spread. This is done in cases where there is a blockage of the bowel; for relieving pressure on the spinal cord which has caused severe pain; or to insert a feeding tube in a patient of oesophageal cancer.

Other forms of surgery performed on cancer patients include **reconstruction surgery**, to restore the body's appearance in case of head or neck surgery for cancers of the mouth, or breast reconstruction after mastectomy. **Prevention surgery** is done for pre-cancerous polyps of the colon, and in women with strong family history of cancer in the breast and ovary, to eliminate their risk of developing the disease in the future. **Laparoscopic surgery** is a minimally invasive procedure performed through small incisions and often robotically assisted in tumours of the chest, prostate, uterus, and ovary. **Laser surgery** focuses high intensity light to cut through the cancer tissue in a precise manner in eye lesions. **Cryosurgery** uses liquid nitrogen to freeze and destroy tumours, particularly in skin and cervical cancers. **Supportive surgery** prepares the patient for chemotherapy by inserting a port through which medication is administered.

Chemotherapy

Chemotherapy is the systemic use of drugs for the treatment of cancer. The main goals of such forms of therapy vary from cure achieved by killing all tumour cells, controlling the growth of cancer cells, thereby causing remission, or palliative care to reduce symptoms and making the patient more comfortable.

Most forms of chemotherapy are administered intravenously. This allows the tumour to rapidly take up the drug, resulting in quick action against the cancer cells which can be present anywhere in the body—be it the site of origin of the tumour or on tumour cells that have spread to distant sites. A single drug, or more frequently, combinations of several drugs that act differently are used to destroy the malignant tumour. Using a combination of drugs reduces the dose of each drug, which is better tolerated by the patient owing to the decreases in their toxic effects. Drug combinations also reduce the chances of developing drug resistance early on (see p. 40 in 'Drug Resistance').

Chemotherapy that is administered before surgery in order to reduce the tumour size is called neo-adjuvant chemotherapy. After surgery, it is designated as adjuvant chemotherapy. The dose of the drug is calculated accurately for each patient, based on either their body weight measured in kilograms or determined by the body surface calculated using the height and weight of the individual.

This form of medication is given in cycles—a dose of the drug followed by several days or weeks without treatment; or it is given for a certain number of days followed by a period of rest; or it is administered every other day for a set number of days, followed by complete rest. The period of no medication gives the body enough time to recuperate from the side-effects on the normal tissues of the body. Some drugs work better when given continuously, while others require three weekly cycles. The schedule for each drug is such that it maximizes the anti-cancer action and minimizes the side-effects. At times, the patient may develop serious side-effects, requiring a change in the chemotherapy plan or even stopping the drug.

The Cell Cycle in Chemotherapy and Radiation

An overview of the cell cycle brings clarity to the way the drugs used in chemotherapy and radiation work, and their effects. The cell cycle is the normal life cycle of a cell.[13] It comprises five phases, out of which G0 is the resting phase.

G0 Phase: Most cells in adults are resting or quiescent, and do not undergo active cell division. To re-enter the cell cycle, the cells must be stimulated by signals. These signals push the cells out of G0 (this phase lasts from a few hours to a few years) into the next phase of the cycle.

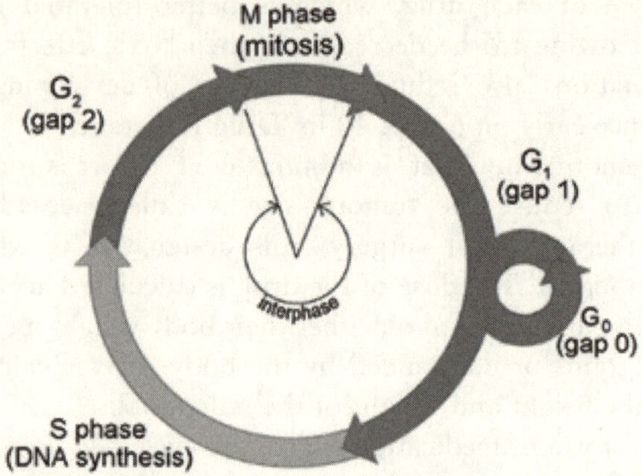

G1 Phase: In this phase (lasting 18–30 hours) the cells begin to grow and become larger in size by manufacturing more proteins.

S Phase: In this phase, the DNA content of the nucleus doubles and the chromosomes replicate to form two copies. This ensures that the daughter cells formed on completion of cell division have matching DNA. It lasts for about 18–24 hours.

G2 Phase: In this phase, further growth of the cell takes place and the DNA is ready to split into two identical cells. It lasts 2–10 hours.

M Phase (mitosis): In this phase, the cells split into two daughter cells. It lasts only 30 to 60 minutes.

An understanding of the cell cycle enables the oncologist to decide which drug, or combination of drugs, are best suited to curtail and destroy the tumour. Most chemotherapeutic drugs work only on cells that are actively dividing. Some drugs specifically attack cells in a particular phase of the cell cycle, either the S phase or the M phase. Cells in the resting phase, or G0, are not targeted by chemotherapy. Based on these facts, the oncologist can plan how often the dose of each drug should be administered for optimizing the beneficial effect of treatment.

Most chemotherapeutic agents, besides being cell-cycle specific, have a dose-related plateau in their cell-killing ability. Therefore, to increase the cell kill, there is a need to increase the duration of exposure, rather than increasing the dose of the drug. As some drugs are phase-specific, attempts have been made to time drug administration in such a way that the cells are synchronized into a phase of the cell cycle that renders them especially sensitive to the cytotoxic agent.

The shorter the cell cycle, and the larger the fraction of cells in the cell cycle at a given time—the more susceptible is the cancer to chemotherapy. Cancer cells grow more rapidly when the tumour is small, and the blood supply can keep pace with its growth. Once the malignant cells outgrow the blood supply, they undergo necrosis or cell death. Dead tissue has poor or no vascular supply—thus any remaining viable cancer cells in the necrotic area are likely to escape being targeted. Chemotherapy, therefore, is most effective in small, rapidly growing tumours.

The drugs used in chemotherapy act in two ways: one, attacking rapidly dividing cells and interrupting the cancer cell cycle by preventing mitosis or cell division; two, by inducing cancer cells to undergo programmed cell death. Drugs used for chemotherapy do not differentiate between normal cells and cancer cells. They target all cells that are in the dividing phase of the cell cycle. In other words, there is collateral damage to some normal cells.

Targeted Therapy

Targeted therapy is a form of chemotherapy given to some patients with cancer. The principle behind targeted therapy is that cells have triggers (molecular targets) on their surface, which receive signals that control their function and determine their growth and proliferation. These triggers have been identified in some types of cancer cells. Targeted molecular therapy is sometimes referred to as 'precision medicine' or 'precision therapy'. It uses information about the genes and proteins of a tumour, not only for diagnosis, but also to treat it. These therapies are the current focus of new anti-cancer treatments.

There are two types of agents used in targeted therapy: one directed against the tumour cells, and the other against the supporting tissue of the tumour. Monoclonal antibodies act against specific triggers on the tumour cells and are an example of the former. Small molecule (anti-angiogenesis) drugs which block the formation of new blood vessels resulting in starvation of the cancer cells is the mode of action of the latter.

TARGETED THERAPY Vs REGULAR CHEMOTHERAPY

- Targeted therapy blocks the specific trigger or receptors on the cell surface of the cancer cell, so that no signal is received by them. These signals are essential for the growth of these cancer cells.
- Malignant cells without the specific triggers are unaffected, therefore, it has little impact on normal cells.
- Chemotherapy, on the other hand, acts in a non-specific way on all rapidly dividing cells, normal or cancerous, in particular phases of the cell cycle and not on any specific target.
- Targeted therapies are designed to interact with specific triggers and are not chosen for their ability to kill rapidly proliferating cells.
- Toxicity resulting from targeted therapy includes skin-related problems like dryness and rashes, delayed wound healing, clotting disorders, and hypertension.

Targeted Therapy in Some Cancers

Breast Cancer: Tissue removed by excision biopsy of the breast is tested for a trigger called Human Epithelial Growth Factor Receptor 2 protein (HER2). When HER2 expression is high on the surface of some breast cancers, targeted therapies can be used to destroy these tumour cells. When malignant cells are negative for HER2, targeted therapy has no role to play.

Melanoma: Some melanomas produce altered proteins that drive cancer progression. The cell growth signalling protein, BRAF (an oncogene) is targeted in its altered form to contain the spread of this form of skin cancer.

Lung Cancer: Drugs that block the Epithelial Growth Factor Receptor (EGFR) can stop or slow the progression of lung cancer positive for EGFR.

Leukaemia: Some chromosomal abnormalities present in leukaemic cells result in the formation of fusion genes, the products of which produce fusion proteins. Fusion proteins are targeted in this form of treatment.

Hormone Therapy: Certain tumours thrive in the presence of hormones. Blocking the hormone receptors stops or slows the growth of hormone-sensitive tumours. Hormone therapy is used in the treatment of breast and prostate cancer.

Radiation Therapy

Radiation therapy is another important localized modality used in the treatment of cancer. It can be used in combination with surgery and/or chemotherapy, or in isolation—depending on tumour type. About 50 per cent of patients with cancer receive radiotherapy. It may be given prior to or after surgery. It is a low-cost alternative in cancer treatment.

How It Works

The basis of radiation therapy is the interaction of ionizing particles with the tissue at the molecular level. The ionizing particles could be x-rays, gamma rays or electrons. This interaction depends on the energy created by the production of the secondary charged particles, usually electrons, which break the chemical bonds within the nucleus and cause irreversible cellular injury and death of the cell.

There are two ways to deliver radiation therapy: external beam radiation or external radiotherapy, along with interstitial implants which require placing radioactive material in the body near the cancer cells, or even a combination of the two. The Linear Accelerator Imaging technology has made radiation therapy extremely targeted and highly effective—permitting delivery of the radiation beam with sub-millimetre precision. The direction and strength of the beam can be individualized for each patient, thereby minimizing the exposure of healthy tissue and related side-effects.

The goal of radiation therapy is to maximize the dose to the abnormal cells while minimizing the exposure of normal tissue. The effects of radiation therapy are not immediate, they generally occur over a period of time. Tumours with rapidly dividing cells respond more quickly to radiation than slowly growing ones. Radiation is painless and does not make the patient radioactive. It may be administered either before or after surgery. When given prior to surgery, it shrinks the tumour and makes removal easier. When given after surgery, it targets any remaining malignant cells at the local site, thus preventing recurrence.

There are three situations wherein radiation therapy is given: as treatment to destroy the tumour and cure the disease, for prophylaxis—to prevent tumours from developing and spreading, as palliative care to relieve symptoms like pain, or for preventing seizures in brain tumours.

How Radiation Kills Cancer Cells

Radiation is a form of localized treatment given to the area where the cancer is located. It kills the cells that are actively dividing, but it is less effective against cells in the resting phase of the cell cycle (G0 cells), or against slowly dividing tumours. The term 'radio-sensitivity' describes the susceptibility of tumour cells to damage by radiation.

Drug Resistance

Hope is being able to see that there is light despite all the darkness.

—Desmond Tutu

How it Occurs

Resistance to chemotherapy is, in many ways, similar to the drug resistance that develops in bacterial infections. It is the innate (or acquired) ability of cancer cells to evade the effects of chemotherapeutics, making it an important problem in cancer therapy and management, as well as affecting a vast majority of patients. Besides, there is no cancer treatment that is effective against widespread disease.

It is important to comprehend that in the process of evolving into a malignant cell, changes take place at the molecular level to immortalize the cancer. To achieve this power of survival and endless growth, the developing cancer commandeers many cellular processes which may ultimately be responsible for drug resistance. It could arise due to host- or tumour-related factors and it is responsible for therapeutic failure—and eventually, death.

Most of the drugs administered do not act to produce their anti-cancer effect just like that. They require activation in the body to achieve potency. Therefore, many host-related factors alter the effectiveness of the drugs by preventing them from reaching their target, rendering them unable to achieve their intended goal. These factors may impact the absorption, distribution, metabolism, or excretion of the drug. They include long-standing toxicity of the drug on the liver and/or the kidneys. The liver is responsible for metabolizing most of the drugs administered and often suffers the brunt of the toxicity, while the kidneys excrete the drug and its breakdown products, which may interfere with its normal functioning.

Failure of the drug's effects can also occur after the drug has reached the tumour. This is referred to as local resistance, and it occurs because the tumour is highly heterogeneous. Heterogeneity implies that one population of cancer cells may be sensitive to the drug, while others may be innately drug-resistant. Chemotherapy kills the sensitive cells, leaving behind a high proportion of drug-resistant cells. These resistant cells have a propensity to grow unhindered while the patient is still on a particular treatment. As time passes, the cancer continues to grow and further treatment with a particular drug is completely ineffective.

In fact, drug resistance is complicated and has many factors. Programmed cell death is promoted by p53—the protector of the genome in response to chemotherapy. But p53 is mutated in about 50 per cent of the cancers, hence this gene is rendered non-functioning and allows drug resistance.

Another factor includes the receptors on the cell surface and the transporter substance within the tumour, which control the entry of the drugs into the malignant cell. Enhanced transporter substances within the tumour cells are associated with poor prognosis due to rapid drug efflux. Inhibitors of these transporter substances are being used in treatment, along with chemotherapy, to reduce drug efflux and increase the concentration of the chemotherapeutic drug within the tumour cells.

It has also been seen that over time, elevation of certain enzymes within cancer cells enhances the detoxification of the anti-cancer drug. This results in reduced damage to the malignant cell, circumventing the effect of the drug. One of the responses to chemotherapy is DNA damage, but there are inherent mechanisms within cells which repair the damaged DNA. Cells with damaged DNA are removed by the body. When this mechanism comes into play, it also results in resistance. Inhibitors of the repair pathway, taken along with chemotherapy, increase the efficacy of the treatment. It can be said that malignant cells are heterogeneous due to 'aberrant DNA repair mechanisms and cell death dysregulation pathways'.[14]

Malignant tumours also have stem cells which can be drug-resistant. These cancer 'mother' cells persist during remissions, both at the local site of the cancer and in the area of metastasis. It is these cells that may be responsible for relapse at either of these sites. As medical understanding of the molecular mechanisms of drug resistance improves, new solutions are being found. However, a lot more research is needed to unravel the entire picture, and drug resistance remains a challenge.

Fighting Drug Resistance

A drug combination is generally used during chemotherapy to reduce the chances of toxicity and the risk of developing resistance early. When a single chemotherapeutic agent is given, it has to be administered in higher doses and therefore, it is more likely to have many side-effects. The other rationale behind giving a cocktail of drugs is that when several agents are administered, they are likely to target different populations of the cancer cells, thereby reducing the total population of tumour cells that are differently mutated. Resistance to one drug is unlikely to result in resistance to the other.

Outcomes of Cancer Treatments

Let your life lightly dance on the edge of Time,
like dew on the tip of a leaf.

—Rabindranath Tagore

Diagnosis, prognosis and treatment are central to the management of cancer patients. There are many factors that influence the cancer prognosis or outcome. Foremost among these is the stage of the disease at the time of diagnosis. The stage indicates the size of the tumour, and how far it has spread to other parts of the body. Other factors that determine prognosis are: the organ where the cancer is located; the grade of the tumour indicative of how closely it resembles the tissue of origin under the microscope; cancer traits as assessed by the pathologist; age of the patient; health of the individual at the time of diagnosis; and the response to treatment.

Based on a combination of these factors, a favourable prognosis is given when it appears that the patient is likely to respond well to the treatment. Conversely, an unfavourable prognosis indicates that the individual is unlikely to show any benefits from treatment. Moreover, prognosis is a prediction based on data and is not set in stone for any given patient. Some tumours have a better prognosis than others. Conventionally, good prognosis has been described for testicular and skin cancers, while it is poor in oesophageal and pancreatic cancers. At times, the presence of certain markers (like Capn-4) on the cell surface of some cancers heralds a poor prognosis.

Disease-free survival is a statistic—it indicates the percentage of patients who can be expected to have no sign of the original cancer after a fixed period of time, following a standard recommended treatment protocol. Depending on the type and site of cancer, this measure may be one, two, three, or five years. This data is based on large groups of patients, and therefore cannot always accurately predict the response of an individual case.

The five-year disease-free survival rate is generally used as a standard way of discussing prognosis, as well as a way to compare the value of one treatment over another. It is an estimate and is expressed as a percentage, based on information gathered on hundreds and thousands of patients with a specific type of cancer. When a five-year survival is expressed as 80 per cent for a given tumour, then it means that eighty out of every hundred patients treated are still alive five years after the diagnosis.

What does the cancer survival rate fail to tell us and how does it impact us? Even though it gives a general idea of what the outcome is likely to be, it is never specific to the individual. It also does not suggest that a patient can expect to live for only five years after stoppage of treatment, or that the cancer has been cured for all time.

If asked, the treating oncologist generally reveals to the patient what his/her prognosis is likely to be, depending on this statistic. Seeking information about prognosis is a personal choice, and patients should decide how much information they require themselves. Being fully informed about the likely course of their disease helps practical planning and making treatment decisions. The likelihood of a good prognosis may encourage the patient to undertake more aggressive options, if available, with a goal of achieving remission. On the other hand, patients with a poor prognosis may instead opt for palliative care.

The concept of cure implies that there is no trace of cancer after the treatment has been completed. It is assessed after a specific time frame using multiple parameters, with help from clinical, radiological and/or pathological means. Within remission, on the other hand, 'complete remission' indicates the disappearance of signs and symptoms, while they are greatly reduced in 'partial remission'. Remission that persists for five years or more may be considered a cure by some oncologists. The persistence of even a few malignant cells in the body, even in a suppressed state, may be the source of recurrence in case of poor nutrition or low immunity.

Another measure of success in cancer treatment is quality of life. Poor health-related quality of life may be due to the symptoms of the cancer, the side-effects of treatment, and, indirectly, due to psychological problems associated with the diagnosis of a potentially fatal condition. Other chronic illnesses may add to the burden even after the cancer is in remission or has been cured.

In India we often use Western statistics to predict the outcome for cancer, not taking into account the many other variables that exist in the Indian scenario. There is an enormous difference in the prognosis among the rural and urban cancer victims. With little or no medical facilities in remote rural areas, patients tend to seek medical help in the late stages of the disease.

In the advanced stages, the treatment objective is to slow down or stop the advancement of the cancer and, thus, to prolong life—even though the cancer cannot be cured. At times, only active surveillance and follow up may be necessary for the rest of the patient's life. Active surveillance is based on the concept that in low-risk cancer like some cancers of the prostate, the patients do not warrant aggressive, immediate treatment; they are given treatment only when necessary. These patients may live a normal life without therapy for a number of years and may die of causes other than the cancer.

Part II

CANCER AND NUTRITION

The Relationship between Cancer and Food

Your diet is a bank account. Good food choices are good investments.

—Bethenny Frankel

Hippocrates, the great Greek philosopher and the father of modern medical science, said 'Let thy food be thy medicine.' Ignore his words of wisdom at your own peril. The body has an inherent ability to heal itself given the right nutrition, proper environment and adequate exercise. A closer look shows that those who ignore this dictum have ailments that stem from wrong eating habits and require serious lifestyle changes. Most of this is factual information, but it needs to be addressed to put extrinsic factors which cause cancer into perspective.

An aging population alone cannot explain the increased incidence of cancer—it afflicts younger adults and many more children today. Forty years ago, as postgraduate students in pathology, we were taught about the rarity of breast cancer in women in their early twenties. At that time we were told: *This case that you're seeing is one you are likely to see once in your career as a pathologist—a once in a lifetime case.* Astonishingly, many more such cases are being diagnosed today. In my last job as a senior consultant in histopathology at a cancer hospital, I reported two cases in one year. A change is certainly taking place. It is believed that in the next ten years, one in two men and one in three women will develop cancer.

We Are What We Eat

Food is the essence of our lives. It is not only fuel for our bodies, but it nourishes us, and helps us grow. Unlike plants that manufacture their own food, we rely either directly or indirectly on plants for our sustenance. The content of our diet determines our wellness and ability to prevent diseases. Unwise decisions about what we eat may cause harm and sickness.

There are many essential dietary factors that boost our immune system and are essential to fight all types of diseases, including cancer. Low immunity is responsible for many illnesses. HIV-AIDS proves this point—it is an acquired infection associated with low CD-4 (a type of lymphocyte) cell counts, and therefore associated with low immunity. Patients with this disease suffer not only from the same type of infections as everyone else, but also from some infections caused by organisms which do not infect healthy individuals. They have an increased incidence for certain cancers as well.

Processed Foods Lower Immunity and Increase Risk of Disease

Omnipresent cancer-causing agents are more likely to cause cancer, in case of lowered immunity. A considerable number of these agents come from the food we eat. Unwittingly, we consume these foods over long periods of time, providing fuel to the developing abnormal cells. By nourishing them and giving them the impetus they need for growth and multiplication, they further mutate and result in the development of cancer, which manifests many years later.

At times, changes take place in our food habits—not all of them for the better. Some of these changes are influenced by factors like poor knowledge of a balanced diet, migration for economic reasons and adapting to the new environment, changes in the pace of life and its associated stresses; and increased consumption of precooked or take-away foods. Changes in dietary habits, fast foods, and obesity contribute to the increased incidence of ill health, and even cancer. It is believed that half of all cancers worldwide are related to lifestyle and poor diet.[15]

Often, urban Indians' nutritional consumption comes from refined sugars, refined flour and vegetable oils. I asked our domestic help, Gita, about the changes in her diet since she moved from the village to the city three years ago. She said that refined sugar or refined flour was almost never consumed by her or her family in the village—it was unaffordable. The tea they drank was black, without sugar. Now, for her a cup of tea (approximately 180 ml) has two and a half spoons of sugar, is whitened with milk, and is consumed twice a day. They have white bread with tea for breakfast—there is no time to make rotis of whole wheat or millets, as all members of the family, including her, work. Evening tea is drunk with glucose biscuits. For her family, an increase in sugar consumption and eating bread or biscuits made of refined flour are signs of prosperity. However, refined sugar and refined flour can cause weight gain and increase the risk of heart disease and diabetes; they are unhealthy choices.

There can be no shortcuts in the preparation of a healthy meal. Pre-cooked food, or food from restaurants may contain flavour enhancers and preservatives, both of which are detrimental to health. Flavour enhancers can cause rashes, headaches, breathing difficulties, sleep disturbances and irritable bowel, while preservatives may cause headaches, palpitations, allergies and even cancer. Besides, the ingredients used in pre-cooked or restaurant food may not always be fresh, and flavour enhancers may also be used to camouflage stale food.

The United Nations has designated the years 2016-2025 as the decade of nutrition.[16] For this initiative to succeed, it is imperative to have knowledge about the foods we eat—which foods contribute positively to health and which are harmful.

The NOVA Food Classification

The NOVA classification of food is centred around the nature and extent of food processing. It is a helpful indicator for the safety of the food we consume. According to the NOVA classification, Group 1 is unprocessed or minimally processed food, while Group 4 relies predominantly on modification of foods to entice customers by making it highly palatable. Such ultra-processed products dominate the food industry in the Western world today. Fortunately, this dominance of Group 4 foods is restricted in India. However, we too are gradually forgetting how healthy our native diet is and are swinging towards Western influences.

THE NOVA FOOD CLASSIFICATION[17]

- Group 1: Foods in this category are either fresh, frozen, or dried. They include fruits; leafy and root vegetables; grains, legumes like beans, lentils, and chickpeas; starchy roots and tubers like potatoes; fungi like mushrooms; meat, poultry, fish and seafood; eggs; milk; fresh fruit or vegetable juices without additives (sugar, sweeteners or flavours); pasta, groundnuts and other oil seeds without added salt or sugar; spices such as pepper, cloves and cinnamon; and herbs such as thyme and mint; plain yoghurt with no added sugar or artificial sweeteners; tea, coffee, drinking water.
- Group 2: These include processed culinary ingredients, i.e. substances obtained directly from Group 1 foods or from nature through processes such as pressing, refining, grinding, milling, and spray drying. Some examples are sugar, salt, molasses, honey, maple syrup, vegetable oils, butter and lard.
- Group 3: These are products made by adding sugar, oil or salt to Group 1 or Group 2 foods. Typical examples

of processed foods are canned or bottled vegetables, fruits and legumes; salted or sugared nuts and seeds; salted, cured, or smoked meats; canned fish; fruits in syrup; cheeses; unpackaged freshly-made breads and alcohol of all types.

- Group 4: The ingredients of these foods are also used in processed foods, such as sugar, oils, fats, salt, anti-oxidants, stabilizers, and preservatives. The main purpose of industrial ultra-processing is to create products that are ready to eat, drink or heat. They are liable to replace both unprocessed and minimally processed foods that are naturally ready to consume such as fruits and nuts, milk and water, and freshly prepared drinks, desserts and meals. Common attributes of ultra-processed products are hyper-palatability and sophisticated, attractive packaging. Examples of typical ultra-processed products are: carbonated drinks; sweet or savoury packaged snacks; ice-cream, chocolate and candies; mass-produced packaged breads and buns; margarines and spreads; biscuits, pastries, cakes, and cake mixes; breakfast 'cereals', 'cereal' and 'energy' bars; 'energy' drinks; milk drinks, 'fruit' yoghurts and 'fruit' drinks; cocoa drinks; meat and chicken extracts and 'instant' sauces; infant formulas; and many ready-to-heat products including pre-prepared pies and pasta and pizza dishes; poultry and fish 'nuggets' and 'sticks', sausages, burgers, hot dogs, and other reconstituted meat products; and powdered and packaged 'instant' soups, noodles and desserts.

Recent ongoing research has furnished evidence that a 10 per cent increase in the proportion of ultra-processed foods in the diet was associated with a significant increase of 12 per cent in the risk of overall cancers, and 11 per cent in the risk of breast cancer.[18] Many hypotheses have been put forward to explain these findings. One suggests that the poorer nutritional content of such diets which are rich in ultra-processed foods, sodium, fats (both total and saturated) and sugar, and poorer in fibre and various micronutrients, contribute to weight gain and risk of obesity. Obesity is recognized as a major risk factor for post-menopausal breast cancer and stomach, liver, colorectal, oesophagus, pancreas, kidney, gall-bladder, endometrium, ovary, and prostate cancers as well as haematological malignancies. This diet is associated with raised blood sugar levels and a lower satiety effect.

Foods preserved with salt and nitrites are associated with an increased risk of stomach cancer. In Western countries there has been a sharp rise in the intake of ultra-processed foods, which make up 25-50 per cent of the daily calorie intake.[19] The materials used in the packaging of such foods—which remain in contact with it—also have carcinogenic and endocrine disruptor properties.

A Balanced Diet

Our food preferences usually dictate our diet. These preferences can be accommodated, provided we strike a balance between the various components of our daily food. Varying the content ensures that the meal is wholesome and tasty at the same time. We must make smart choices by rationalizing what we eat and in what combination. For example, a combination of potato curry and rice, or potato curry and puri, amounts to eating starch with starch, leading to a higher risk of diabetes, heart disease and obesity.

Variations in Diet Can Affect Incidence and Types of Cancers

The varying frequencies of different tumours across geographical areas has been attributed to the variations in diet among the people living in different areas. For example, the incidence of colon cancer in Japanese men and women in the age group of fifty-five to sixty years was negligible fifty years ago, when compared to those in the US or UK. However, studies have shown a progressive increase in colon cancer in the Japanese population that moved from Japan to Hawaii and from there to mainland America.[20] This was attributed to the 'Americanization' of the healthier Japanese diet. The reverse is also true, with the incidence of stomach cancer, which was high in the native Japanese population, reducing in the second generation Japanese whose parents had migrated to the US.

Another example can be seen from the betel chewing habit prevalent in India, which is responsible for the high incidence of mouth cancers in this country. There are many ingredients, including tobacco, which act in concert to produce these cancers. Individually, the ingredients are weak carcinogens, however, chewing paan or paan masala every day over prolonged periods of time is extremely harmful. Indians living abroad who have no access to paan and have given up this habit, have a lower chance of developing these cancers.

There are many types of diet. To facilitate understanding of the strengths and weakness of a diet in relation to longevity, I have listed a few, along with the diseases most commonly associated with each.

The Indian Diet

The geography of India is varied, including a large coastal belt, landlocked plains and mountainous areas. Where we live influences our food habits, as do local customs and practices. Fish is eaten more frequently in the coastal belts, while more chicken or meat is consumed inland. In north India wheat and millets are the staples, while in the south and east of the country they are rice and millets.

Though the composition of the food eaten varies according to the state, it is largely vegetarian. Even when meat, poultry or fish are eaten, they are only consumed in small quantities. The usual meal comprises of rice or roti eaten with dal (lentils) and/or subzi (vegetables) and dahi (homemade yogurt). These are healthy food habits, but many types of deep-fried snacks, better classified as 'Indian junk food', are often consumed between meals. Potatoes are another junk staple: it is not uncommon to eat a meal of potatoes with rice or Indian breads, and they are often used as fillers to bulk up vegetables. Indian sweets, nothing but concentrated sugar, are also consumed in large quantities.

Even the cooking medium differs across various states and depends on the local plant source. Coconut oil is used in Kerala, sesame oil in other southern states, mustard oil in the north and east of the country and peanut oil in central India, while urban areas use sunflower, soyabean, hydrogenated vegetable oils, butter and ghee.

Pickles and chutneys are also eaten with every meal. Interestingly, spices are grown mainly in south India, and the food there tends to be spicier. Indian food is generally rich in carbohydrates, sugar and salt. This type of diet is associated with hypertension, obesity, diabetes and heart disease. Cancers of the mouth and throat, and those related to obesity are common.

The Western Diet

Often referred to as the 'meat and sweet' diet, the typical American diet is rich in saturated fats, red and processed meats, refined carbohydrates, junk food (or fast food), and is loaded with sugar and salt. The food may contain preservatives and food colouring. It is low on fresh fruits and vegetables, whole grains and seafood. Sausages, burgers, salami, cheese, industrial yogurt, French fries and high-sugar drinks are commonly consumed. Hamburgers with

French fries, for example, make up a meal rich in fat, including cholesterol and carbohydrates, and low in fibre. The ill-effects of these include hypertension, heart disease, diabetes, obesity and colorectal cancer. It is the diet chosen by many people in developed countries, and increasingly, in developing countries as well.

The Mediterranean Diet

The Mediterranean diet is an example of healthy eating—rich in vegetables and fruit, whole grains, legumes, nuts and fish. Healthier fats such as olive oil replace butter. Herbs and spices are used for seasoning rather than salt. This type of diet is associated with a reduced risk of death from heart disease as well as from cancer.

The Japanese Diet

The Japanese have one of the longest lifespans in the world. Their diet is known to be the healthiest, based on the large variety of vegetables, tofu and fish it contains. However, in some areas it is high in salted foods and is associated with a high rate of infection with *H. pylori*—a bacterium known to contribute to cancer of the stomach. This, in fact, is the commonest type of cancer seen in Japan. The wide variety of mushrooms which are part of this diet are known to have a protective effect against stomach cancer.

When comparing all the diets mentioned above, it would appear that the Mediterranean diet is possibly the healthiest, while the Japanese have a diet that promotes longevity.

Diet-related Risk Factors in Cancer Development

The impact of food in the development and progression of cancer, though documented, is not entirely, comprehensively understood. Nevertheless, it is crucial to examine the evidence, particularly since the toxic substances in our food are often without odour, colour and taste. Therefore their presence is hidden from us and we only become aware of them once cancer develops and we analyze our food habits.

Foods that Cause Cancer

Some known cancer-causing substances like the following may exist in our food. The following is by no means a comprehensive list:

- Aflatoxin is present in peanuts and rotten grain, and causes liver cancer.
- Food additives (monosodium glutamate, artificial food colouring, sodium nitrite) and artificial sweeteners (aspartame, sucralose and saccharin) may cause bladder cancer.
- Pesticides in fruits and vegetables may be responsible for cancers of the breast, prostate and brain. High levels of pesticides have been found in apples, pears, peaches and grapes, and also in green vegetables like spinach, mustard, and lettuce. Washing or peeling may reduce the level of these pesticides, but since some of them are resistant to breakdown, some trace amounts remain in our food.
- Other foods like farmed fish which are fed farm waste may also be rich in pesticides and other harmful chemicals.
- Oestrogen-like chemicals—xenoestrogens—from herbicides and pesticides attach to and accumulate in the fat cells of farm animals. Certain plastics that are by-products of industrial waste may contain xenoestrogens.
- **Refined carbohydrates** in white bread, cakes, pasta and sweetened juice are low in fibre, vitamins and minerals. Besides, they raise blood sugar levels rapidly. High-blood sugar acts on the immune system, reducing the protective phagocytic activity

of the white blood cells (cells that engulf ineffective organisms and destroy them), and thereby decreasing the individuals' ability to fight against infections or even destroy cancer cells. Blood sugar levels above 120 mg sustained over a period of time substantially reduce the body's ability to fight infections.[21]

- At times, cancer-causing substances are synthesized in the stomach from the food we eat. Nitrosamines cause gastric cancer.[22] These may be produced by the digestion of proteins, or from preservatives used in food, or through the reduction of nitrates found in common vegetables to nitrites. Processed meats contain sodium salts of nitrates and nitrites as preservatives, which increase the risk of colon cancer. Deep frying at high temperatures also produces nitrosamines.
- Experiments on animals fed genetically modified (GM) foods have shown a greater risk for cancer development.[23] GM plants have their DNA altered in a way that does not occur in nature. Proponents of GM products consider them safe, but further testing may be required. Genetic modification is done to increase the yields of farm crops for instance, by increasing the herbicidal tolerance of plants. Its impact on humans is the subject of ongoing research. It is believed that, like pesticides, herbicides and fungicides are substances that mimic oestrogens. Xenoestrogens, as mentioned earlier, play a role in the development of breast, prostate and brain cancers. These hormones and hormone-like substances act by attaching themselves to cell surface receptors, triggering a chain reaction which stimulates growth of the epithelial cells, which may ultimately result in cancer development.
- BT corn is genetically altered to express one or

more protein of the bacteria *B. thuringiensis*. These bacterial proteins are poisonous to particular insects that attack the corn. Such corn, expressing the bacterial proteins that repel the insects, when consumed by humans, can interfere with the normal bacterial flora of the gut and may replace them with harmful ones. The normal flora are vital for a healthy body and play an important role in fibre digestion and the synthesis of certain vitamins.

- Sugar substitutes like aspartame[24] and saccharin, and food additives present in soft drinks and processed food, are carcinogenic in animals.[25] Monosodium glutamate (MSG) added to enhance the flavour of processed food is also carcinogenic. Aspartame and glutamate (excitotoxins) damage the nerve cells by excessively stimulating them.
- Synthetic emulsifiers are in use in a wide variety of processed foods, even in cakes, biscuits and ice cream. Though FDA-approved, animal experiments with some emulsifiers like carboxymethyl-cellulose and polysorbate 80 have shown that these may interfere with gut mucus resulting in the bacterial penetration of the epithelium, thereby producing low grade inflammation and metabolic syndromes.[26]

Alcohol

It is often advised that one should drink less to reduce the risk of cancer. Ethanol or ethyl alcohol, the chemical substance found in beer, wine and liquor is produced by the fermentation of sugar and starch by yeast and belongs to Group 3 in the NOVA classification of foods. The content of alcohol in each of these drinks varies from 3 to 7 per cent in beer to 35-40 per cent in distilled spirits like gin, rum, vodka and whiskey. Alcohol is catalyzed by alcohol dehydrogenase and aldehyde dehydrogenase in the liver.

Ethanol is eliminated from the body through its oxidation first to acetaldehyde and then to acetate. Ethanol, *per se*, is not mutagenic, but acetaldehyde, the product of broken down ethanol, is carcinogenic and mutagenic, binding to DNA and protein. Thus, alcohol generates reactive oxygen species that damage DNA and lipids by oxidation, and increase the blood levels of oestrogens, besides impairing the body's ability to break down and absorb nutrients like vitamins A, B complex, C, D, and E. Apart from these, alcohol may contain carcinogens as contaminants introduced during fermentation, like nitrosamines, phenol and hydrocarbons.

The American Society of Clinical Oncology (ASCO) considers alcohol a modifiable risk factor for multiple malignancies caused by excessive long-term alcohol consumption. Minimizing excessive alcohol intake has 'important implications for cancer prevention'.[27] For example, in 2012, 5.5 per cent of all new cancer occurrences and 5.8 per cent of all cancer deaths worldwide were estimated to be attributable to alcohol.[28] Alcohol consumption is causally associated with oropharyngeal, laryngeal, esophageal, hepato-cellular, breast, and colon cancers.

Alcohol may be a risk factor for other malignancies, including pancreatic and gastric cancers. When alcohol and smoking are combined the risk of cancer increases manifold.

Post-menopausal women with a high daily intake of alcohol are more prone to develop cancer than non-drinkers. Additionally, the liver damage caused by alcohol interferes with the detoxification of hormones, resulting in increased levels of oestrogens in the blood. The end result is an enhanced incidence of breast cancer.

Foods that Help Against Cancer

Numerous naturally occurring protective factors are present in the food we eat.

The most prominent of these is **fibre**, which is preventive against colon cancer. High-fibre content in the diet is also responsible for slowing down the absorption of natural sugars. Lower blood sugar levels result in better functioning of the immune system. The fibre we eat feeds the millions of bacteria that live in a symbiotic relationship in our intestine—keeping both the mucosa and the cells of the immune system in a state of good health.

The Importance of Fibre in Our Diet

Fibre in the food is something that the body needs but never actually digests. It comes in two forms: soluble and insoluble fibre. Most plant-based foods have a mixture of both. The soluble fibre turns into a gel in the stomach and slows digestion. This helps in lowering cholesterol and blood sugar after a meal. Insoluble fibre, on the other hand, remains as such, all the way to the colon, making the waste heavier and softer and easier to evacuate. The increased intestinal bulk decreases transit time, which in turn decreases the exposure of the intestine to harmful substances that may be present in the food.

These non-digestible carbohydrates are ultimately fermented in the colon by anaerobic bacteria to Short Chain Fatty Acids (SCFA). These fatty acids stimulate the colonic epithelial cells to multiply, producing anions (negative charged ions) that serve as nutrients for the mucosal cells, stimulating their growth by improving their blood flow. The healthy supply of mucus creates a protective layer that shields the mucosa and prevents the bacteria from getting too close to the intestinal epithelial cells. Research done in the last decade has made it apparent that these fatty acids are key to the prevention of obesity, inflammatory bowel disease and colonic cancer by maintaining a normal gut bacterial flora.[29]

In addition, there are anti-bacterial molecules present in the mucus the keep the bacterial flora in check. This results in a peaceful coexistence between the bacteria, epithelial cells of the colon and the immune system. This fibre, though undigested by the human body, is digested by the gut bacteria that break it down through their enzymes to produce waste matter. Recent research suggests that some SCFA may be absorbed and travel to other organs, in particular the lungs.[30] The bronchial mucosa is rich in mucus-producing cells, thereby modulating the immune system there. It can, therefore, be said that a diet rich in fibre impacts the lung functions positively.

A diet high in fibre can prevent re-absorption of substances that have been excreted in the bile from the intestine. In the absence of enough fibre, re-absorption of hormones or drugs back into the circulation results in prolonging their effect on the body, which is, at times, harmful. Taking the example of oestrogen, which has a distinct role in the development of breast cancer, it was observed that in pre-menopausal women given a diet of low fat and high fibre, there was little or no effect on the total circulating oestrogen.[31] However, there was a significant reduction in the most potent female hormone—oestradiol. This reduction persisted over time while the women remained on this diet.[32]

Fruits and vegetables like guava, pears, banana, beetroot, peas, carrots, turnip, eggplant, cabbage, cauliflower and broccoli, besides all types of nuts, are rich in fibre.

Micronutrients: Important Vitamins and Minerals

Micronutrients consisting of vitamins and minerals that are required daily, though only in small quantities. These are essential for human development and in the regulation of normal metabolism.

- **Folic acid** belongs to the B-complex group of vitamins, occurring naturally in green leafy vegetables like spinach, and is often present in manufactured fortified foods like cereals, milk, fat, oil and infant formulae. Folic acid has a distinct cancer-fighting ability. Research on smokers consuming recommended daily doses of 400 micrograms of folic acid has shown their risk of developing pancreatic cancer reduced by almost half.[33] Folic acid prevents DNA mutations which occur because of smoking, toxins, pollution and radiation. During cell division, adequate amounts of this vitamin ensure that DNA replication occurs in an orderly manner. Low folic acid level in the blood is also associated with anaemia.

- It is an established fact that **Vitamin D** or the 'sunlight vitamin' is fat soluble and is essential for the growth and strength of bones and teeth. Besides this, research has suggested that it has strong anti-cancer properties, curbing the growth of cancer cells.[34] Improving **calcium** and Vitamin D nutritional status substantially reduces all cancer risk in post-menopausal women. Vitamin D regulates the expression of more than 200 genes involved in cell proliferation, cell differentiation, formation of new blood vessels and programmed cell death. Low levels of this vitamin are associated with an increased incidence of breast, colon and prostate cancers.
- Lung cancer patients treated by surgery had higher survival rates in summer than in the winter months because Vitamin D is readily generated in the skin in the summer. Doses of 1,000 international units (IU) of Vitamin D are recommended for both men and women. Good sources of Vitamin D are **milk, sea food (cod, shrimp and salmon), eggs and sunshine.** Exposure to ten minutes of sunlight generates 5,000 IU, if 40 per cent of the body is exposed (without sunscreen, of course).
- Minerals are micronutrients necessary for the

proper functioning of the body. These include **iron,** calcium, **zinc, magnesium,** and selenium. **Selenium,** along with **vitamins C, E** and **beta-carotene,** blocks chemical reactions that create free radicals in the body. Micronutrients prevent damaged DNA molecules from replicating, thus preventing cancer from developing. They also make chemotherapy safer. **Mushrooms, egg yolks, sea food, meats, garlic, onions and broccoli are rich sources of selenium.**

Obesity and Cancer

The Definition and Spread of Obesity

Obesity is the condition where an individual has an excessive proportion of body fat. The Body Mass Index (BMI) is a common method of accurately measuring obesity. BMI is measured by dividing the weight in kilograms by the height in meters squared (see box for values). Compared to normal persons, those who are overweight or obese are at greater risk of impaired health. Obesity carries a higher risk of diabetes, cardiovascular disease, strokes and cancer. In simple terms, it is a caloric imbalance occurring when the intake of calories is far in excess of the actual requirement of the body.

BMI calculator

BMI	BMI Categories
Below 18.5	Underweight
18.5 to 24.9	Normal
25.0 to 29.9	Overweight
30.0 or >30	Obese

Obesity is an ever-increasing epidemic, resulting in a substantial public health crisis in many countries, as the numbers of obese individuals steadily increase. A survey done in the US in 2015–16 showed the prevalence of obesity as 39.8 per cent in adults and 18.5 per cent in youth (below nineteen years of age). Obesity was higher among middle-aged adults (forty–fifty-nine years) at 42.8 per cent when compared to young adults (twenty–forty-nine years) at 35.7 per cent. The incidence of obesity was higher among children between six and eleven years (18.4 per cent) and adolescents between twelve and nineteen years (20.6 per cent), as compared to children aged between two and five years (13.9 per cent).

Obesity is caused by certain lifestyles, which can include a lack of physical activity, smoking and drinking, as well as a diet rich in processed foods. Till recently, obesity was a major health problem in developed countries, but now this problem is surfacing in developing countries like India. The relationship between obesity and cancer strongly suggests that eating a healthy diet and controlling body weight is an established method of preserving good health.

Obesity Causes Cancer

Many cancers, including those of the oesophagus, liver, kidney, pancreas, breast, uterus, colon, thyroid and gall bladder are related to obesity. **Being overweight increases the cancer risk by 40 per cent for some types of cancers, which is higher than the cancer risk associated with smoking.**[35] Both men[36] and women[37] with high BMIs (greater than 25kg/m^2) have higher incidence of cancer.

In addition, obese patients with cancer have poorer outcomes, increased risk of recurrence and overall increased mortality. This is true for both men and women. Weight loss after the diagnosis of cancer, in an overweight individual, improves the survival rate.[38]

Many mechanisms have been suggested to explain the development of cancer due to obesity:

- Increased synthesis of the female hormone, oestrogen, from precursors in the fat cells of the body has been seen in obese women. The increased risk of post-menopausal breast cancer is thought to be linked to increased levels of oestrogen in these women.
- Apart from this, there is an increased incidence of Type 2 diabetes in obesity. Obesity produces hyperinsulinemia and insulin resistance with insulin-like growth factors which promote tumour formation. Diabetes is associated with chronic infection and higher blood sugar. Both factors that play a role in tumour development and progression by interfering with the normal functioning of the immune system—reducing the ability of the white blood cells to swallow and kill infectious agents like viruses, bacteria, and fungi.

Weight Loss Reduces Cancer Risk

Numerous observational studies have examined the relationship between weight loss and cancer risk and results suggest a decreased risk of breast and colon cancer among individuals who lose weight.[39] Strong evidence suggests that patients who undergo bariatric surgery to lose weight had a lower rate of obesity-related cancer than those that did not.

Preventing obesity by consuming a diet low in animal fat and rich in vegetables, with adequate exercise, may be the answer for maintaining good health and impeding the development of cancer.

Cumulative data collected over the last thirty years on diet, physical activity and weight control has established, without a doubt, a link between lifestyle and cancer. Clear-cut recommendations on reducing cancer risk have become a project in cancer prevention. This 'blueprint', if followed closely, will reduce the risk of developing cancer.

Recommendations for Cancer Prevention

New reports from the World Cancer Research Fund (WCRF) 2018 and American Institute of Cancer Research (AICR), in a continuously updated project, review the role of diet, physical activity and cancer.[40] They highlight that no single factor is responsible for reducing cancer risk. It is the diet and lifestyle patterns working together that can increase or decrease the cancer risk. The cancer prevention recommendations from the report are:

1. Maintain a healthy weight throughout life (during childhood, adolescence and adulthood). The report provides evidence that body fatness and cancer risk has grown stronger both for adulthood and childhood obesity.
2. Physical activity has a protective effect against several cancers. It should be moderate, limiting sedentary habits which favour obesity.
3. Eat a diet rich in whole grains, vegetables, fruits, pulses and lentils. The food should have at least 30 grams of fibre daily, avoiding starchy vegetables and fruits.
4. Limit intake of fast food and processed foods high in fat, starch and sugar. This helps maintain a healthy weight and prevents obesity.
5. Limit the consumption of red meat and processed meat.
6. Limit the intake of sweetened drinks, drinking mostly water and unsweetened drinks. Sweetened drinks are linked to childhood obesity.
7. Limit alcohol consumption as far as possible. For cancer prevention, it has been suggested that one should avoid alcohol.
8. Do not use supplements for cancer prevention. All nutritional needs should be met through diet alone.

9. Breastfeeding is good for mother and child, protecting mothers against breast cancer and children against childhood obesity.
10. Cancer survivors should follow a diet that fulfils their nutritional needs following the guidelines for cancer prevention, and indulge in regular physical activity.

MAINTAINING GOOD HEALTH THROUGH DIET

- Eat a balanced diet rich in vitamins A, C and E, and minerals like calcium, magnesium, iron, zinc, potassium, sodium, chloride, iodine, selenium and fluoride.
- Boost the immune system by eating vitamins E and D, as well as turmeric.
- Eat yogurt to maintain the normal gut bacteria essential for proper digestion of food.
- Give up tobacco chewing or smoking—this is associated with a significant drop in the risk for cancer.
- Limit the amount of refined sugar and white flour in your food—these are pro-inflammatory, cause hyperinsulinemia and release an insulin-like growth factor.
- Limit the consumption of margarine, animal fat and vegetable oils rich in omega-6.
- Choose leaner protein sources such as fish, low fat dairy products, lean meat and chicken. Meats, cheese and butter are rich in saturated fats, and are associated with obesity—an important predictor of cancer. Red meat consumption should not exceed 300–500 gm per week.
- Avoid processed meats. Sausages and bacon can be eaten very occasionally—eating them daily as a breakfast staple is a no-no. Smoked meats are rich

in nitrites and nitrates—these preservatives increase the risk of stomach cancer.

- Alcohol should be avoided in excess, as it is associated with an increased risk of cancer of the mouth, breast and oesophagus. Do not exceed more than one drink a day for both males and females.
- Avoid fast foods.
- Avoid sugary drinks. Eat energy-dense food sparingly.
- Avoid salty food, pickles and preserves.

Using the Beneficial Effects of Food in Cancer

> *To all the beasts of the earth and all the birds in the sky and all the creatures that move along the ground—everything that has breath of life in it—I give every green plant for food. And so it was.*
>
> —Genesis 1: 29-30 (NIV)

The beneficial effects of food can be maximized by manipulating the contents of our diets. In other words, we can use nature to stabilize our bodies. Unlike genetic factors, diet is easily modifiable and can therefore alter the cancer risk. Foods can fight infections, improve immunity and elevate mood—doing it all naturally. A large amount of data has established that eating certain types of foods regularly may have a preventive role in cancer development.[41] Second, once cancer has developed, it is possible that consuming these foods may help us recover from the disease as well as from the effects of treatment.

This is a bit like exercise—thirty minutes daily improves life-expectancy by 50 per cent. A 2012 report from the American Cancer Society strongly suggested that diet, exercise and weight control increases survival time, and could even keep us cancer-free.[42] Exercise keeps weight in check and increases circulation, resulting in the removal of toxins that may have accumulated. It also improves mood and sleep, besides reducing anxiety.

Recent data coming out of King's College, London, suggests that exercising sufficiently as we age prevents the immune system from declining and protects the elderly against infections.[43] The benefits of exercise are reflected both in the body and mind, maintaining the muscle mass and propping up the immune system. The immune system is at its functional peak at age twenty, following which there is a slow but steady decline—which is why the elderly are susceptible to infections, rheumatoid arthritis and even cancer. It was observed that non-competitive endurance cycling, even in the elderly, produced high levels of T cells (a type of lymphocyte that is protective against infection and cancer)—almost as much is produced in a twenty-year-old—thereby providing protection against these ailments.

Foods to Fight Depression

The World Health Organization (WHO) rates depression as a 'significant contributor to the global burden of disease' in the Western world, i.e. predisposing us to many other diseases.[44] It is characterized by a general feeling of being low, loss of appetite, disturbed sleep and an agitated state of mind. It can be considered both as the cause and as an effect of cancer. The question then arises: can diet play a role in mood elevation?

Yes, it can. Serotonin is a neurotransmitter (a chemical messenger that transmits signals from one nerve cell to another) responsible for the proper functioning of the brain. It maintains equilibrium in the brain cells. Its absence affects appetite, mood, sleep pattern and sexual desire. A drop in serotonin levels may be one of the causes for depression. There are certain types of foods that are rich in serotonin—they are nature's antidepressants.

L-tryptophan is an amino acid that boosts serotonin levels in the blood and subsequently in the brain. It is present in **whey protein, cottage cheese, eggs, sesame seeds, oats, mangoes, bananas, bread, pasta, sweet potatoes, walnuts, chickpeas,** and **poultry**. Other natural antidepressants include **Omega-3** (abundant in **fish** like **salmon, sardines, mackerel,** and in **flax seeds**); **vitamin B6, B12** and **folic acid**; and **vitamin D** (the sunlight vitamin), which is produced in the skin from cholesterol. In winters, inadequate sunlight interferes with the formation of vitamin D and therefore, depression usually worsens during these months, particularly in the Western countries. Finally, balanced blood sugar levels are necessary for proper functioning of the brain. Any fluctuation in blood sugar is considered the single most important factor in mood disorders.

Foods to Boost the Immune System

For our fight against cancer, the immune system is vital. It's efficient functioning determines the state of our health. It defends the body against pathogenic organisms like bacteria and viruses, and removes both dead and abnormal cells. Immune system dysfunction due to poor nutrition is associated with increased risk of infection. Simply put, proper nutrition gives fire power to the defending army—the immune system.

To slow or even stop the progress of cancer requires galvanizing the immune system. This will clear the inflammation and remove the mutated abnormal cells. If the cancer has established itself in the body and treatment is essential, the revitalization of the natural defence mechanism of the body becomes crucial to fight the cancer. A multi-pronged attack including the activated immune system, surgery, radiation and/or chemotherapy is most likely to beat the odds.

The immune system has two components: soluble antibodies and cellular components like lymphocytes and macrophages to fight infection and remove damaged tissue generated in the process. The tissues most exposed to pathogenic organisms are the skin and the intestine. These are the body's natural barriers, separating us from the world of pathogens outside. Both these tissues are rich in immune cells which can further signal recruitment of other similar cells when the need arises.

These barriers are kept in perfect health by the food we eat. Supportive foods are **vitamin A, B, E** and **C**, and food containing **fibre**. Fibre in the food is fermented into SCFA in the large intestine. This nourishes the colonic mucosal lining, and adds bulk to the intestinal content, removing toxins and waste matter by ensuring complete evacuation. The body's dietary requirement of fibre is 20–30 grams per day.

Foods rich in **proteins, antioxidants, essential fatty acids, vitamins** and **minerals** keep the immune system in perfect health. **Eggs, fish, tofu, nuts, leeks** and **green vegetables** provide the daily requirement of these essentials. **Fruits** and **vegetables** rich in antioxidants boost the immune system. On the other hand, processed foods and food contaminated by pesticides or toxic metals like lead and mercury are immunosuppressive. Some food additives, particularly, emulsifiers like lecithin used to keep water and oil mixed in margarine, baked foods and ice cream, destroy vitamins like B1, C and E present in the food and depress immunity. Mono and diglycerides used in peanut butter act similarly.

Link between Immunity and Depression

There is a link between neurotransmitters released in response to emotions and the activity of the immune system. Natural killer cells (NK cells) are lymphocytes that can directly destroy tumour cells, and are the first line of defence against cancer. They were found to be more active in women with breast cancer who could better face the disease psychologically than in those who sank into depression.[45] In another study about women with ovarian cancer, it was found that those who felt loved and supported, with higher morale, had better functional NK cells, compared to those who felt depressed, alone and abandoned.[46] There is truth in the expression that the battle against cancer, like all battles, is won and lost in the mind.

Ketogenic Diet and Fasting

The ketogenic diet has been used in the past as a therapeutic tool. This diet has a fat content of 90 per cent, moderate to low proteins of 8 per cent, and very low carbohydrates, comprising 2 per cent of the total calorie intake. The ketogenic diet was found to be beneficial for epilepsy, when followed for short two to three weekly courses. Recently, it has been used as an adjuvant (accompaniment) to chemotherapy. Its most publicized success comes from a report of two women with advanced malignant brain tumour, where their tumours regressed by 21 per cent while on the ketogenic diet.[47]

THE KETOGENIC DIET

- **Breakfast**: eggs with or without bacon.
- **Lunch and Dinner**: tuna salad/grilled fish/ tandoori fish/ mincemeat cutlets/ shell fish/ poultry served with cheese/paneer and lentils. All cooking is done in butter.
- **Vegetables** served with the meal are green beans/ spinach/lettuce/broccoli/cauliflower/bell peppers.
- **Snacks**: Nuts and seeds in full cream yoghurt or berries of various types served with cream.

How It Works

The rationale behind this diet is minimizing the carbohydrate intake and replacing it with healthy fats and moderate amounts of protein. Normal cells of the body have the metabolic ability to adapt from using glucose to using ketone bodies for their energy requirements. Ketone bodies are breakdown products of fatty acids—they are produced in the liver during periods of starvation or while on a carbohydrate restrictive diet. Cancer cells lack this ability to metabolize ketone bodies and, as a result, they are effectively starved.

Additionally, the lipid metabolism—the breakdown of fat—in a ketogenic diet forces normal cells to derive their energy from mitochondrial metabolism. But since cancer cells have dysfunctional mitochondria, they face further stress, being unable to utilize ketone bodies, which results in cancer cell death. Proponents of the ketogenic diet have labelled cancer as a mitochondrial-metabolic disease. The mitochondria are the power generators of the cell and can be damaged by inherited mutations, or by environmental factors and toxins. The last word on this type of diet has not been written; though understandably, it is difficult for patients to follow.

Fasting is akin to a ketogenic diet and it has been found to enhance the responsiveness of chemotherapy and radiotherapy. Fasting cycles are reported to retard tumour growth in non-diabetic patients.

Methods of Cooking in the Fight Against Cancer

Cooking methods vary—some are healthier than others. Generally, slow cooking or cooking at lower temperatures is an ideal way to cook. Sound methods (requiring little to no extra oil or fat) include the following:

- baking and oven roasting;
- braising or browning ingredients first in a pan, then cooking covered with small quantities of liquid;
- steaming, which requires the ingredients to be placed in a perforated utensil over simmering water;
- sauté-ing or stir-frying which uses small amounts of oil while stirring constantly till the vegetables are cooked.

Cooking methods that should be avoided are broiling and grilling thin pieces of meat exposed to direct heat over a charcoal grill or direct flame. All high-temperature cooking produces chemicals like heterocyclic amines and polycyclic aromatic hydrocarbons that are known carcinogens. Microwave cooking in a microwave-safe dish involves rapid cooking at high temperatures—although it uses less oil, it is a questionable method because of the high temperatures attained.

Recommendations on Carbohydrate, Protein and Fat intake

Plants

The key strategy in using food for cancer protection is based on harnessing the plants' own mechanisms of self-preservation—used against fungi, bacteria and insects—to protect ourselves. Unlike animals, plants are unable to move away from the pests that attack them so, over time, they have developed many safeguards for their survival. If plants are eaten in their natural form they lend these protective effects to humans.

While there is no single plant that can keep us cancer-free, combining many types of fruits and vegetables, with their different defence abilities acting synergistically, could be hugely beneficial. Thus, a well-oiled immune system can prevent the cancer cells from taking root. Additionally, eating the right quantities of food in order to maintain a healthy weight is equally important. Knowledge and its implementation are central—recognizing the protective effects of the various types of food adds a new dimension to eating.

Meats

Urbanization and economic prosperity has increased the demand for meats. One of the commonest red meats eaten in India is mutton. Both goat meat and lamb are referred to as mutton. Goat meat is the healthier of the two. The other common meats consumed are chicken, beef and pork.

Chicken farms are not always hygienic—birds are seldom free range, they are often kept in crowded coops to increase production, fed a diet to rapidly enhance growth, and given antibiotics to prevent infection. On the other hand, goats are free-range and graze on fresh vegetation. **Goat meat** is lean and easy to digest, contains high potassium content and is low on sodium, when compared to other meats. Goat meat is high in HDL (good cholesterol) and low in fat and LDL (bad cholesterol). In fact, it has the lowest number of calories in comparison to beef, chicken, pork or lamb. Three ounces of goat meat (about 90 grams) has 122 calories, while chicken has 162. Pork has the highest calorie content.

Carbohydrates

Of the daily caloric requirement, 45–65 per cent should come from carbohydrates. The body has a carbohydrate reserve in the form of glycogen stored in the liver and the muscle—this helps maintain normal blood sugar levels. In the absence of adequate carbohydrate intake, glycogen from the stores is broken down, first, to provide for the energy needs of the body. This is followed by the breakdown of amino-acids from the muscle, resulting in loss of muscle mass, and the breakdown of fats resulting in weight loss.

Proteins

Of the daily caloric requirement, 10–25 per cent should come from proteins. They provide amino-acids which are the building blocks for tissue repair, hormone and enzyme synthesis, and for maintaining the immune system. Animal sources of protein are high in saturated fats and have no fibre or vitamin C. Plant proteins, on the other hand, from grain and legumes, contain both fibre and vitamin C.

Sattu is a drink made from the flour of roasted gram and, at times, of roasted barley. It is a poor man's super food. It is drunk as a sherbet by body builders, gymnasts and wrestlers after a full workout. It has 20 per cent protein by weight and is a good source of iron, calcium, manganese and fibre and is easy to digest. It is consumed in Bihar, Punjab, Utter Pradesh, West Bengal and Madhya Pradesh, either as a drink or as stuffing in roti or puri, or as litti chokha (sattu stuffed ball of flour baked in a coal fire). The protein content of sattu is equivalent to that of whey. It is considered effective in osteoporosis.

Recipe for Sattu Sherbet: 1 cup water, 1½ tablespoons of sattu, pinch each of black salt, roasted cumin seed powder and ½ teaspoon lime juice. Mix well and drink.

Fats

Fat intake should not exceed 30 per cent of the daily caloric intake. Fats are essential for maintaining the cells, skin and hair, for hormone synthesis, and for providing the body with fat soluble vitamins (A, D, E and K). Surplus calories consumed are stored in the body as fat. Fats contain fatty acids. The source of fat may be animals or plants. Animal sources are rich in saturated fats while vegetable oils contain unsaturated fats as well.

Fatty acids

There are two essential fatty acids required by the body, since these are not manufactured by us. They are derived from the diet and include **alpha-linolenic acid (omega-3)** and **linoleic acid (omega-6)**. Omega-3 and omega-6 are important for the normal functioning of all tissues of the body. Adequate intake of these fatty acids results in many health benefits. The main advantages of these essential fatty acids are that they maintain the health of the cardio-vascular system, help foetal growth, proper growth and development of children, brain development, and pain relief.

Omega-3 has a crucial role in cancer prevention and

possibly, cancer cure. The ratio of omega-3 to omega-6 in the diet should be 1:1 or higher.[48] A higher ratio is associated with lower risk of breast cancer.[49] For this reason, it is best to avoid diets that are rich in oils, consisting of processed foods—these are high in omega-6 but low in omega-3. Though both omega-3 and omega-6 are found in fruits, vegetables, nuts, seeds, vegetable oils and legumes, the richest sources of omega-3 are **flax seeds, canola, walnuts** and **soya bean. Fish** is another good source of essential fatty acids. However, it is also rich in cholesterol, and may contain toxins if the water they breed in is contaminated.

Cooking Oil

It is often advised that more than one type of oil should be used as a cooking medium, depending on the dish or the method of cooking. Oils with a more balanced ratio of **omega-3/omega-6** are more suitable, like **light olive oil** and **flax seed oil**. Other oils, like canola, are high in omega-3 but canola is sourced from genetically modified seeds, which need further testing. Sunflower oil has a high smoking point, is rich in vitamin E but contains only omega-6. Coconut oil is rich in saturated fats and raises total cholesterols. **Peanut oil** is a good all-purpose oil. Mustard oil contains erucic acid and is banned in the US and Europe because it causes nutritional deficiencies and heart lesions in animal experiments. **Rice bran oil** has a high smoking point and is high in unsaturated fats and antioxidants.

The decision of selecting a cooking medium is influenced by many factors besides taste preferences:

- Firstly, the content of saturated, poly-unsaturated and mono-unsaturated fats in the oils. Unsaturated fats eaten in moderation and replacing saturated or transfats can help lower cholesterol and risk of heart disease.

- Secondly, a high smoking point, since at this point a lot of nutrients are lost and some foods become potentially harmful with the formation of aldehydes, which are toxic for the liver.
- The process used for the extraction of oil is crucial. Cold pressed oil is extracted at low temperatures with no loss of nutrients; using an expeller and squeezing is superior to chemical extraction.

The emphasis should be on increasing plant and animal sources of omega-3 in the diet and decreasing sources of omega-6. Omega-3 inhibits Cox-2 enzymes, which are pro-inflammatory and harmful to the nuclear membranes of cells, while omega-6 is pro-inflammatory. This may play a role in malignancy as chronic inflammation is linked to cancer. The role of Cox-2 inhibitors is an area of active research in cancer therapy. Colonic cancer is associated with high levels of Cox-2 in 85 per cent of the cases. In a study of breast cancer it was found that women who were cancer-free had higher levels of omega-3 in their breast tissue. Similar findings were reported for prostate cancer. Other compounds that inhibit Cox-2 enzymes are **aspirin, aloe vera, ginger, garlic and turmeric.**

Recommendations: Corrective Dietary Measures

The preferred environment of developing cancer cells differs from that of normal healthy cells. When the environment is perfect, it provides all the ingredients that are conducive to cancer growth, allowing them to behave like parasites. The trick is to disrupt their preferred environment.

Where normal cells derive their energy from carbohydrates in the presence of oxygen, cancer cells produce energy in the absence of oxygen. This anaerobic type of metabolism which takes place within tumour cells maintains an internal milieu of low pH in which cancer cells thrive. Therefore, both factors—low oxygen levels and low pH—are pro-cancer factors as they promote the growth of tumour cells. Some studies have shown that a high oxygen tension of 95 per cent is lethal for cancer cells, without any effect on normal tissues. This is the rationale behind the use of hyperbaric oxygen for treating cancer.

On the other hand, eating a diet rich in carbohydrates results in the sugars being rapidly broken down by cancer cells in the absence of oxygen to produce lactic acid—the resultant low pH promotes tumour growth.

Having understood that cancer cells have traits that can be countered by the diet, the corrective measures that need to be introduced into the diet are two-fold: first, remove harmful substances from the daily foods and second, introduce foods that have a protective effect.

Removing Harmful Substances from Our Diet

a) At the individual level:

Giving up smoking or chewing of tobacco are proven methods for the prevention of some types of cancer. Likewise, reducing the intake of refined sugar, white flour, and fat—which are pro-inflammatory, low in fibre, and promote obesity—reduces the incidence of colon cancer. Avoiding cakes, Indian sweets, chocolates, fizzy drinks, sugary tea and processed foods can help. Common salt can cause an oestrogenic effect on the cells. WCRF states that both salt and salt-preserved foods are associated with an increase in the risk of stomach cancer.[50] Therefore, all processed, canned food, dried salted meats, sausages, pickles and Chinese food rich in MSG should be avoided.

b) At the agricultural level:

Better regulation of the farming sector may pay dividends. Organic farming relying on fertilizers such as compost manure, vermi-compost, green manure and bone meal, with restrictions on synthetic fertilizers and pesticides may go a long way in improving the safety of food. Once the crop is harvested, proper storage and a good delivery system is required.

Fruits are generally picked slightly raw when they are firmer and easier to transport. However, their natural ripening process, which is slow and associated with a change of colour, softening of texture and the development of fragrance, is hastened through carcinogenic artificial agents (compromising on the colour, taste and fragrance). Calcium carbide is the most commonly used artificial ripening agent in India. It is banned in many countries as it is a known carcinogen and contains traces of arsenic and phosphorus, making it a health hazard. For artificial ripening, packets of calcium carbide are placed in the box containing the fruit. In the presence of moisture from the fruit, acetylene gas is generated, which is similar to ethylene—a natural ripening agent produced by the fruit. This compound is used by retailers to ripen bananas, mangoes, jackfruit and litchi.

Introducing Foods that Have a Protective Effect

Foods can act indirectly against cancer through their anti-inflammatory and mood elevation effects, as well as directly, by preventing new blood vessel formation, providing antioxidants and stimulating the immune system. Cognizance of these anti-cancer properties can lend our diet a (cancer) preventive role.

Using these protective aspects, I have divided food according to their most potent properties into four main groups: anti-inflammatory, antioxidants, stimulants of the immune system, and anti-cancer. However, there may be considerable overlap in these groups as some foods provide multiple safeguards, including additional properties like anti-depressant effects and their vitamin and fibre content.

Foods with Anti-Inflammatory Effects

It is an established fact that chronic prolonged inflammations may progress to become cancer over time. Consuming foods that have anti-inflammatory effects turns the clock back and causes healing, preventing cancer formation. Foods rich in anti-inflammatory substances are **turmeric**, **pulses**, **cruciferous vegetables** and **citrus fruits**.

Home remedy for chronic inflammation: ½ teaspoon of turmeric powder in 1 teaspoon of honey and a pinch of pepper.

I am reminded of a friend who was being treated for breast cancer when she developed skin-related problems after treatment. She had an embarrassing itching on the head and neck. Her CBC (complete blood count) was normal but the ESR (erythrocyte sedimentation rate: a nonspecific measure of inflammation) over the past six months had remained high. Her treating doctor had prescribed an anti-histamine to be taken whenever the symptoms were severe. Over dinner one evening, the discussion shifted to home remedies for chronic inflammation. I mentioned having read about turmeric, **honey**, and **black pepper** working wonders in such conditions. She took it for twenty days then rang to say her itching had subsided without the anti-histamine. A month later her ESR had dropped by 30 per cent.

Turmeric is a rhizomatous herbaceous perennial plant belonging to the ginger family. People say that turmeric powder adds flavour to food and years to your life. Indian foods invariably have significant amounts of this spice. In South Asia it is used in cooking almost all types of vegetables, lentils, rice and meats. Turmeric interferes with the cell signalling pathway, stopping cells from progressing into tumours, suppressing their further growth and their ability to spread locally. The molecule responsible for this anti-cancer effect is curcumin. Laboratory evidence suggests that it inhibits the growth of tumours of the colon, liver, breast, stomach and ovary.[51]

The main mechanisms of turmeric's anti-tumour effects are its powerful anti-inflammatory action, prevention of new blood vessel formation, forcing cancer cells to self-destruct, and enhancing the effect of chemotherapeutic drugs when administered. This is responsible for the lower rate of cancers of the colon, breast, and kidney among Indians when compared to the West, despite the greater exposure to uncontrolled environmental carcinogens in India.[52] Black pepper is added for better absorption of curcumin from the diet. Black pepper contains piperine, which enhances the bio-availability of nutrients absorbed by the body. Piperine increases the bio-availability of curcumin almost twenty-fold.

Citrus fruits like **oranges, grapefruit, lemons** and **sweet lime** contain anti-inflammatory **flavonoids**. These are potent detoxifiers of carcinogens in the liver. The largest amounts of flavonoids are present in the peel of the citrus fruit.

Foods with Antioxidant Effects

These include **tea, pulses, spices, cruciferous vegetables, garlic, berries, tomatoes, grapes, peanuts** and **grain**. Antioxidants prevent oxidative stress, which is a disturbance in the balance between the production of reactive oxygen species and the body's antioxidant defence. Reactive oxygen species are free radicals that contain one or more unpaired electrons, because of which they are highly unstable (or 'reactive'). In order to stabilize themselves, they attempt to steal electrons from other molecules, leading to injury of cellular components such as DNA, proteins or lipids. Antioxidants, conversely, are molecules that are capable of donating electrons to the free radicals without being destabilized themselves. An imbalance between oxidants and antioxidants is the underlying basis of oxidative stress.

Many conditions arise due to oxidative stress, including Parkinson's disease, Alzheimer's, gene mutations, cancer, cardiovascular disorders and inflammatory diseases.

Teas of all types, produced from the *Camellia sinensis* plant, are rich in **polyphenols**—a class of antioxidants that scavenge for cells damaged by free radicals in the body and detoxify them. These are ten times more potent than antioxidants found in any other fruits or vegetables. Although there are iced teas and instant ready-to-drink teas, it is the brewed hot tea (green, black or oolong tea) that has the higher concentration of polyphenols, while decaffeinated tea has lower levels.

In India, **tea** is a staple. It is mainly drunk hot. It is believed that three cups of tea neutralizes free radicals, while three to five cups a day can stop the growth of certain cancers, particularly, breast and prostate cancers. Increased sugar consumption associated with tea-drinking can be avoided with unsweetened tea.

In animal experiments, antioxidants induce death in tumour cells and block tissue invasion by cancer cells. They hinder cancer's growth, prevent new blood vessel formation (necessary for tumour progression), protect the skin against damage by UV light, and modulate the immune system. Laboratory tests using **catechin**—an antioxidant found in tea—have substantially slowed tumour cells of kidney, breast, prostate, and skin cancers as well as leukaemia. When green tea is combined with radiotherapy, the effect of treatment is enhanced in brain tumours.

Spices are a ubiquitous ingredient of Indian food. The variation in the ingredients used is responsible for the difference in taste in every home. In India, there is no such thing as 'curry powder'—a legacy that the British carried back with them, which is still available in England. In fact, in a traditional Indian home it is not unusual for the spices to be freshly ground or pounded every morning, according to the requirements for the day. Generally, there are no premixed 'masalas'. The rationale behind the use of basic spices is to use the combination best suited for your palate. Also, prior mixing of spices may cause some interaction between them, changing the taste and causing loss of flavour.

Allspice or *kabab chini,* also known as Jamaica pepper, gives the flavours of cinnamon, nutmeg and cloves although it is a single spice. It is used in making meats and desserts. It has anti-microbial, antioxidant, anti-cancer and analgesic properties, thanks to the presence of flavonoids, phenolic acid and catechins.

Basil, originally native to Iran and India, has antioxidant, anti-bacterial and anti-mutagenic properties due to components like **linalool, cineole, estragole** and **eugenol.**

Cardamom is a common ingredient of Indian cooking. It has antioxidant properties.

Coriander is native to Southern Europe, North Africa and South Asia. Although all parts of the plant are edible, its fresh leaves and dried seeds are most frequently used in cooking. It is a common ingredient in many foods throughout the world. One of its principal constituents is linalool, a potent antioxidant.

Cumin is native to the Eastern Mediterranean region and India. **Thymoquinone** (TQ) is its active ingredient which exhibits antioxidant, anti-microbial and anti-inflammatory properties. TQ is effective in cancers of bone, ovary, colon, breast, leukaemia and pancreas.

Whole grains: Grains have been a part of the human diet for thousands of years. Rice originated in India. To begin with it was eaten in the wild form but, somewhere, over time it evolved into the more presentable, polished and fragrant version which makes for the exquisite presentation and taste of pulaos and biryani. However, nutritionally rice lacks many vitamins, minerals and fibres. All the nutrients are lost in the process of milling, along with the husk, bran and germs.

Refined flour entered our diet similarly. It is rich in simple carbohydrates with no fibre or vitamins, and is associated with heart disease, diabetes and cancer. Apart from wheat and rice, which are generally consumed more in urban areas, grains like **bajra, jowar, ragi, buckwheat, corn** and **barley** are commoner in rural India. **Whole grain** has three components: bran, germ and endosperm. Whole grain and **unpolished rice** provide the most health benefits. Though the use of multigrain flour has gained popularity, eating flour from a single whole grain at a time, and cycling through a variety of individual grain flours, possibly provides the goodness of all the different varieties of grain—besides being easier on the digestive system.

Epidemiological studies have found whole grains to be protective against some cancers, especially in gastrointestinal cancers and hormone-dependant cancers, including breast and prostate cancers.[53] Whole grains are a rich source of carbohydrates, proteins, fibres, antioxidants, trace minerals, phenolic compounds and vitamins. The phenolic compounds are antioxidants having a cancer-preventive role. Whole grains have a significant amount of **phytoestrogens** that are considered protective in hormone-dependent cancers. Additionally, grains are rich in fibre and contain fermentable carbohydrates that produce SCFA—a source of energy and protection for cells lining the colon.

Foods that Stimulate the Immune System

Many types of foods stimulate the immune system to function better, thereby improving the internal defence mechanisms of the body (immune surveillance) and checking the mutated abnormal cells from taking root. Mutations occur due to several reasons like injuries caused by toxins, oxidative stress, chemicals or radiation. The strongest argument in favour of immune surveillance is the increased frequency of cancers developing in immune-deficient individuals. A weakened immune system promotes cancer. It therefore becomes imperative to strengthen immunity to beat the cancer. Exercise and a balanced diet act as immunity boosters. Foods that stimulate the immune system are **nuts, garlic, mushrooms, fish** and **dairy products**.

Mushrooms belong to the fungus family. Some edible mushrooms include shiitake, kawaratake, maitake and cordyceps. They have cancer fighting ingredients, as do, to a lesser extent, the common button mushrooms. Mushrooms have been staple foods in China, Japan and Korea for many centuries and their consumption in these cultures has been associated with disease prevention and treatment, besides longevity. They contain a molecule called lentinan which, along with other polysaccharides present in these fungi, stimulates the immune system directly. Mushrooms have also been found to be anti-oxidant, anti-diabetes, anti-cancer, anti-allergic and anti-microbial.[54]

Evidence from the same study suggests that patients with colon cancer, who ate mushrooms during and after chemotherapy, lived longer and had a better quality of life. This was true for ovarian, gastric, colon, breast and lung cancer. Trials conducted using the most potent immune-supportive agents extracted from mushrooms showed a distinct role in cancer prevention and cancer treatment.[55] Mushrooms compliment not only chemotherapy but also radiotherapy by countering the side-effects commonly seen in these treatments, such as nausea, bone marrow suppression and anaemia. Some mushroom extracts have been combined with anti-cancer drugs and work in synergy as effective tools in the treatment of drug-resistant cancers.[56] A WHO report suggests that the new drugs that are being developed do not necessarily eradicate tumours but when combined with other agents may turn fatal cancers into manageable chronic illnesses.[57]

Fish are a rich source of proteins, vitamins and long

chain omega-3. Long chain omega-3 is a powerful anti-inflammatory substance. Omega-3 helps restore the length of the telomeres of chromosomes, a property that increases longevity. Vitamin A in oily fish helps fight cancer. The richest sources of vitamin A are mackerel, herring and salmon. Fish oil reduces the rates of breast, colon and prostate cancers.

Milk, yoghurt, butter and **cheese** are commonly consumed dairy products. These are rich in saturated fats, proteins, calcium and fat-soluble vitamins. Skimmed milk, low in saturated fats, is better than whole milk. Butter and cheese have well balanced omega-3 and are better than margarine. Milk derived from cattle that have been administered hormones to improve yields is definitely harmful for humans. Milk that is free from hormones is not associated with an increase in incidence of breast carcinoma in post-menopausal women.[58] Pre-menopausal women with a high intake of low-fat dairy products were also found to have reduced risk of breast cancer.[59] The same study found a similarly inverse relationship between breast cancer and calcium and vitamin D (components of dairy products).

Lactobacillus, the active culture of bacteria in yogurt helps fortify the immune system. The lactobacilli are a part of the good bacteria normally present in the gut. Plain yogurt is better than flavoured products with high sugar content. The regular inclusion of yogurt in the diet increases the internal production of interferon—a powerful cytokine used by the immune system against tumour cells—by three times. Yogurt has been shown to activate natural killer cells and it slows the growth of cancers of the gastrointestinal tract. It also plays a role in lowering cholesterol levels in the blood.

Foods that Are Directly Anti-Cancer

Some foods act directly on the cancer cells—blocking their growth, preventing angiogenesis (the formation of new blood vessels to feed the growing tumour), promoting them to self-destruct, blocking androgen/oestrogen receptors, or even modifying cellular detoxification processes. Many spices, pulses, nuts, seeds, vegetables and fruits fall into this category of foods directly negating the cancer cells.

Cinnamon is a spice obtained from the bark of an evergreen tree belonging to the *Lauraceae* family. Major constituents in cinnamon include cinnamaldehyde, eugenol, and terpinene. Half a teaspoon of cinnamon powder eaten daily significantly reduces the risk of cancer. It is a natural food preservative and a source of iron and calcium. It reduces tumour growth and prevents new blood vessel formation. The ability of cinnamon extracts to suppress the in-vitro growth of *H. pylori*, a recognized risk factor for gastric cancer, gastric mucosa-associated lymphoid tissue lymphoma, and pancreatic cancer, has stirred considerable interest in the potential use of this spice.

Cloves are flower buds of the *Eugenia caryophyllata* tree. Several bioactive components are found in cloves, including tannins, terpenoids, eugenol, and acetyleugenol. Though native to Indonesia, cloves are used in cuisines throughout the world. Studies conducted in mice suggest its effectiveness, especially in modifying cellular detoxification processes.[60]

Cayenne peppers and **red/green chillies** contain **capsaicin** which is known to destroy prostate cancer in mice.

Saffron is a spice derived from the flower of the *saffron crocus*, a plant native to Southwest Asia. Saffron contains more than 150 volatile and aroma-yielding compounds. A carotenoid called crocetin is responsible for its rich golden-yellow colour and is the primary cancer-fighting substance.

Pulses are a staple food in India. **Lentils, chickpeas, beans** and **soya** are a great source of fibre and proteins. In fact, they are the main sources of proteins for vegetarians. Unlike animal protein, they do not contain saturated fats, but they do have fibre. Pulses contain **phytochemicals.**

When consumed in adequate quantities, phytochemicals reduce the risk of cancer. Their protective effect is seen in most types of cancers, predominantly due to their anti-inflammatory effects. Epidemiological data supports this link, but more clinical studies are required. The anti-cancer effect is attributed to its various components like **inositol** and **pentakisphosphate** which block tumour growth and enhance the effects of other treatment. According to one study, eating **beans** three times a week reduces the risk of colon polyps (pre-cancerous lesions) by one-third.[61] Both fibre and antioxidants in beans are responsible for the anti-cancer effect.

For **soya** and **soya supplements**, opinions diverge with respect to breast cancer—from being helpful, to having no effect, to being downright harmful. Soya foods have **isoflavones** which are plant-based, weak oestrogen-like compounds. Breast cancer is an oestrogen-driven tumour. Oestrogen promotes the development, growth and spread of the disease. Therefore, opinions differ on the use of soya products.

Phytoestrogens are plant-based compounds that can activate oestrogen receptors in the body. They are endocrine-disruptive (they interfere in endocrine functions). Therefore, they can either reduce oestrogen activity by blocking the individual's more potent oestrogens from binding to the receptor or lead to increased oestrogen activity by activating the receptors.[62] Oestrogens are a family of hormones—some are weak, like oestrone, while others are strong, like oestradiol. Plant oestrogens, on the other hand, are far weaker than the oestrogens naturally occurring in women, but they can still block the receptors effectively, preventing oestradiol from getting attached. Phytoestrogens are much weaker than the oestrogens present in our body. They block the oestrogen receptors on the cancer cell and slow the growth of hormone-driven cancers.

Proponents of soya products support this view. The jury is still out on the role of soya products in breast cancer. But some studies suggest the use of soya products as a natural alternative to oestrogenic drugs to relieve symptoms of menopause.[63] However this use is controversial as the risk outweighs the benefits. If soya products are consumed throughout one's life, they possibly yield greater benefits than when one's intake starts at menopause. It is also suggested that there may be a difference in the impact of these isoflavones in different racial groups.

Nuts and **seeds** are a great source of vitamins, minerals, proteins, fats and fibre. Opinions differ on the effectiveness of each nut, therefore the best strategy is eating a combination daily. Almonds, walnuts and pecans lower cholesterol and help in fighting cancer. Cashews are rich in tryptophan which works as an anti-depressant. Flax seeds are a good source of omega-3, even better than fish oil. Apricot seeds are bitter, but contain B17, which may have strong anti-cancer properties.

Fruits and **vegetables,** specifically cruciferous vegetables or members of the cabbage family including **cauliflowers, cabbages, broccoli, Brussels sprouts, collard greens** (haak), **bok choy, radishes,** and **turnips** have a promising role in prostate and colon cancer. Their modes of action are multiple: they help protect cells from DNA damage, deactivate carcinogens, have anti-viral and anti-bacterial effects, and prevent angiogenesis. These vegetables contain glucosinolates which are broken down into a number of chemicals that have anti-cancer properties. Some of these are anti-androgens, which prevent proliferation of prostate cancer cells, their consumption being associated with lower cancer rates. Others affect oestrogen metabolism and promote cell death in breast, uterus and colon cancers.

Animal experiments on mice grafted with human prostate carcinoma have shown tumours shrinking to half their size within one month in animals fed these vegetables.[64] Similarly, mice genetically engineered to develop inherent colon polyps at high risk of evolving into cancer, developed half as many polyps as expected when fed **sulforaphane**—an antioxidant released while chewing cruciferous vegetables. The protective sulforaphane is released when the vegetables are cut and chewed. Stir fried or raw in salads is the most effective way to eat them. Broccoli is the most abundant in antioxidants—it boosts the body's cancer protective enzymes, and flushes out cancer-causing chemicals.

Carrots, apricots, peppers and **pumpkins** contain anti-cancer carotenoids like beta-carotene. This is easily converted to vitamin A when required by the body. Raw carrots are rich in pectin which helps healthy gut bacteria to thrive.

Ginger is an aromatic rhizome native to China which has been used as a medicinal plant for many centuries. Its anti-cancer properties are due to many polyphenolic compounds that it contains. Ginger is used along with garlic in cooking many Indian vegetables and meats. It works directly on cancer cells, causing apoptosis (or cell death) induced from within the cells. The main chemo-sensitizing effects of ginger are in ovarian cancers. It selectively kills ovarian cancer cells that have acquired resistance to standard chemotherapy. It destroys cancer cells through two distinct cell death pathways—apoptosis (programmed cell death) and autophagy (self-enzymatic digestion).

Garlic prevents the formation of nitrosamines, a carcinogen formed in the stomach. Food preservatives like nitrates are converted into this carcinogen. Foods rich in garlic reduce the risk of colon cancer in women when compared to those who ate no garlic.[65] Garlic can be eaten crushed or chopped, which helps release the active substances. Garlic contains selenium-, tryptophan- and sulphur-based active agents that attack cancer cells and prevent them from multiplying.

Tomatoes are used extensively in Indian foods. They are

eaten raw in salads, used to garnish lentils, for enhancing the flavours of vegetables and in meats. Tomatoes are a rich source of **lycopene**, a carotenoid responsible for its red colour and which has been found to stop the growth of the cells of endometrial cancer. Other cancers where it has been found to be effective are those of the lung, prostate and stomach. Raw tomatoes have less lycopene, and cooking them provides greater benefits as heating releases increasing amounts of this compound—making more available for absorption.

Berries of all types—blueberries, blackberries, strawberries, and raspberries—are packed with phytochemicals with cancer-fighting properties. In particular, they have high concentrations of phytochemicals called ellagic acid. They are also rich in vitamins C and E, manganese and fibre. Ellagic acid is present in the seeds and people who consume food rich in this anti-cancer compound are three times less likely to develop cancer.[66] They slow the growth of pre-malignant cells and prevent angiogenesis—an essential prerequisite for tumour nourishment, growth and spread. Berries fight colon, oesophageal, oral and skin cancers.

Chlorophyll is the pigment found in green plants which is used to produce food in the presence of sunlight and carbon dioxide. Animal experiments suggest that chlorophyll has a unique anti-cancer property—detoxifying carcinogens like polycyclic aromatic hydrocarbons (generated by incomplete combustion of fuels), aflatoxin (peanuts and poorly stored grain) and heterocyclic amines (grilled meats) in the food. The chlorophyll binds to the carcinogens, thereby reducing its bioavailability. The beneficial effects of eating dark green leafy vegetables like spinach, kale, wheat grass and lettuce is to ensure that the carcinogens remain unabsorbed and are readily excreted by the body. Apart from this, there are other health benefits provided by these green vegetables—fibre, vitamins and minerals.

It is amazing how we have plundered and destroyed our natural environment. We have destroyed nature's green cover by felling trees. We have over-populated her with ourselves, at the expense of her other creatures. We have overfished her seas. We have tried to destroy her ozone layer and polluted her atmosphere. And yet, the earth and nature have stood steadfast in our hour of need, through sickness and cancer she has tried, like a true mother, to provide all the ingredients that may help us heal.

Three Essentials for Good Health

- Balanced diet
- Regular exercise
- Weight control

AN IDEAL DAILY DIET

- 2 ½ cups of fruit and vegetables each day, including citrus fruit, dark green and yellow vegetables.
- High fibre food like whole grain bread and cereal.
- Preferably bake, braise or stir-fry meals to decrease the amount of fat per meal.
- Limit the intake of meats to thrice a week.
- Choose low-fat dairy products.
- Avoid processed food, pickles, Indian sweets and deep-fried foods.
- Limit the intake of alcohol.

Surgery and Nutrition

Your illness does not define you. Your strength and courage does.

—Unknown

Nutrition is an important aspect of cancer treatment at all levels. Eating well, during and after surgery, allows the body to cope better and stay stronger throughout further course of treatment. Good nourishment reduces recovery times. At times, if the patient is underweight, she is put on a diet with more caloric and protein content prior to the surgery, in particular for stomach, mouth and throat cancers.

Post-Surgery Diet and Recovery

Once the surgical part of the treatment is completed, the patient gets a little respite from further treatments till the stitches are removed and the wound has healed. During this period, the food requirements of the patient are **adequate proteins, vitamins and minerals** to enhance healing, to replenish the blood lost during surgery, and to rebuild the immunity and provide the building blocks for tissue repair. In other words, first healing, and then preparing the body for the further onslaught of chemotherapy and/or radiation therapy.

The additional food requirements to hasten repair and healing after surgery focus on increased intake of proteins for repair; vitamin C and other vitamins for wound healing; iron, B12 and folic acid for blood replenishment; carbohydrates and fats for the body's normal energy requirement; and foods for proper functioning of the immune system.

Proteins

Surgery places a considerable burden on the body and an

increased demand for certain foods. Proteins provide amino acids—the building blocks for tissue repair and for keeping the immune system healthy. After surgery, other treatment modalities like chemotherapy and radiation therapy also require extra protein intake. These can be derived from **fish, egg whites, chicken, lean meat, low fat dairy products, legumes like beans and peas and lentils, and protein supplements.** Animal sources of protein are rich in vitamin B12, an essential ingredient for the formation of red blood cells.

Vitamin C

Perhaps the most important nutrients post-surgery are vitamins and minerals. Vitamin C or ascorbic acid is a water soluble vitamin found in a variety of vegetables and fruits. It is a potent antioxidant that protects against free radical injury to the cells. Surgical wounds heal by scar formation. Scar tissue is rich in collagen, which over time matures into fibrous tissue. Vitamin C has a distinct role in collagen synthesis and in the strengthening of the freshly-laid-down fibrous tissue. Deficiency of Vitamin C is associated with delay in wound healing, rupture of the wound and late recovery.

Good sources of Vitamin C are **amla, guava, green leafy vegetables, broccoli, tomatoes, sweet potatoes, berries, citrus fruit, mangoes, red bell peppers, fortified cereal, and the freshly blended fruit juice of any of the above fruits.** The daily requirement for this vitamin goes up from 90 mg for men and 75 mg for women to 500mg or more after surgery. Vitamin C also protects against heart disease by decreasing bad cholesterol, aiding absorption of iron, and supporting the health of the immune system.

Juicing and Blending

The basic principle of juicing or blending is drinking what you cannot eat and giving a headstart to your day with a natural burst of vitamins and minerals. Unlike juice from freshly-pressed fruits and vegetables, packaged juices bought over the counter have exorbitant amounts of sugar and no fibre. Blending is even better than juicing—it pulverizes the fruit or vegetable at high speed so that it retains all the fibre content of the original fruit or vegetable. However, it is important to remember that absorption is quicker after juicing (because of lower fibre content) when compared to a blended drink.

Juice Recipes

For each of the following, blend the ingredients and add 60-90 ml of water, if necessary.

<u>Vegetable Juice (Green Juice)</u>

- 2 carrots
- 10-15 roughly chopped spinach leaves
- 2-3 celery stalks/2-3 amla
- ½ cucumber
- Juice of ½ lime
- ¼ teaspoon olive oil
- ¼ cm ginger

<u>Fruit Juice</u>

- 2 carrots/½ cucumber/1 small beetroot
- 2 oranges
- 1 apple
- ¼ cm ginger

Other Vitamins

Other vitamins that play an important role are:

- Vitamin A: Found in **oranges, green vegetables and carrots**, it promotes wound healing.
- Vitamin D: Found in **milk, fish, eggs and sunlight,** it is a mood elevator and essential for bone repair.

- Vitamin E: Found in **vegetable oils, nuts, liver, milk and eggs,** it protects the body from free radical cell injury.
- Vitamin K: Found in **green leafy vegetables, fish, liver, and oils,** it is necessary for blood clotting.

Iron- and Folic Acid-Rich Food

Surgery is invariably accompanied by some blood loss, which varies with the type of procedure. Haemoglobin is the protein in the red blood cells that carries oxygen to the tissues. The oxygen is necessary for cellular metabolism and healing after surgery. Since cancer cells thrive in anaerobic conditions, adequate oxygenation of blood is anti-cancerous. Consuming iron-rich foods like **liver, meats, clams and green leafy vegetables like spinach,** optimizes the haemoglobin levels and replenishes the iron stores.

Red blood cell formation or erythropoiesis requires iron, folic acid, and vitamin B12. The deficiency of folic acid and vitamin B12 impairs DNA synthesis in the red cell precursors, causing them to self-destruct (apoptosis). This is often referred to as 'ineffective erythropoiesis'. Folic acid is poorly stored in the body and needs constant replenishment. **Many foods contain folic acid, like spinach, sprouts, broccoli, beans, peas, chickpeas, kidney, liver and potatoes.** These should be consumed in adequate quantities after surgery.

Carbohydrates and Fat Requirements

Carbohydrates are the body's major source of energy, providing the fuel for physical activity and for proper organ function. The best sources of carbohydrates are **whole grains, fruits and vegetables.** These foods also supply vitamins, minerals, fibre and phyto-nutrients to the body. Adequate carbohydrate intake in the form of whole grain bread or roti, brown rice, oatmeal and unpolished rice should be ensured. Complex carbohydrates provide nutrients and fibre. Sugar and refined flour should be avoided or restricted. Surgery is accompanied by inactivity, which promotes constipation. Sufficient fibre intake increases the bulk of the intestinal content and reduces constipation. Healthy fats from **olive oil, low fat butter, nuts and seeds** provide the energy levels required after surgery.

Food for Proper Functioning of the Immune System

A properly functioning immune system prevents wound infection and enhances healing. Foods rich in antioxidants, essential fatty acids, vitamins and minerals keep the immune system in good health. Foods that provide us with our daily requirement of these substances are **eggs, fish, tofu, nuts, leeks and green vegetables.**

Food for Mood Elevation

Surgery and hospitalization can be depressing. Engaging the patient in all types of activities keeps them occupied and helps them deal better with their situation. Mood elevators in foods are **fish, flax seed, beans, broccoli, nuts, cereals and banana**. Daily exposure to sunlight also helps in keeping the mood uplifted.

Wheatgrass

Wheatgrass is the stem of wheat seven to ten days after germination. It is believed to possess therapeutic, healing properties. Like most green plants, it is rich in chlorophyll, amino acids, minerals, vitamins and enzymes, and is gluten-free. It can be consumed as a drink.

Wheatgrass is an antioxidant and has anti-inflammatory properties. Other effects include combating anaemia, detoxification by easing constipation through its high fibre content, and stimulation of the thyroid.

Proponents of wheatgrass support its use during chemotherapy. However, there are those who believe that **fresh**

sprouts are far more beneficial than wheatgrass. Sprouts are better tolerated by some patients who have an altered taste—a side-effect of medication. Green juicing—using a range of fresh vegetables—is considered superior to wheatgrass by some. To maximize benefit, wheatgrass could be alternated with green juice.

Wheatgrass Juice: For fresh wheatgrass, blend 3-4 tablespoons of chopped grass in one glass of water. One can also use dried wheatgrass powder—mix one tablespoon in enough whole-wheat flour to make two rotis

Suggested Menu to Promote Healing after Surgery

Once oral feeds are permitted, and there is no restriction on diet, regular food with normal quantities, as per the patient's taste can be provided:

Begin the Day with a Juice

- For juicing, a **mixture of two fruits and a vegetable is ideal** (try **3 oranges, 1 apple and 2 carrots**). The consistency is that of a smoothie. It should not be strained and should be drunk with no additional additives.

Breakfast

- One whole egg and white of second egg (scrambled) with two slices of multigrain bread OR 2-3 cheelas (6") OR 2-3 dosas (6") OR a bowl of cereal with milk, 1½ teaspoon of ground flax seed, 1 tablespoon of chopped walnuts and a sprinkling of cinnamon.
- One cup of tea/coffee with no additives.

Lunch

- Start with mixed vegetable salad.[67]
- Dal
- Two vegetables (for methods of cooking see p. 74 in 'Using the Beneficial Effects of Food in Cancer'). It is recommended that potatoes not be eaten along with rice or chapatis, since that doubles the starch intake and increases the risk of cardiovascular disease.
- Two chapatis (approximately 40-50 gms of wheat flour each) OR rice.
- Curd (60–80 ml), and a fruit.

Tea

- A cup of tea and a tablespoon of a mixture of nuts (almonds, pine nuts, cashew nuts and pumpkin seed).
- Fruit if desired.

Dinner **(Vegetarian/non-vegetarian versions of Indian/Western diets are both possible)**

- Start with a salad
- Meat/fish/chicken/dal (for methods of cooking see p. 74).
- Vegetables (no potato)
- Roti/rice/bread.

After Dinner

- A cup of tea.

Chemotherapy and Nutrition

Life is not a matter of holding good cards, but of playing a poor hand well.

—Robert Louis Stevenson

Before the start of chemotherapy, patients must be taken into confidence about the nature of treatment and its side-effects. This encourages better understanding of this form of therapy and helps patients and caregivers cope better with the side-effects.

Combating the Side-Effects of Chemotherapy

I am reminded of an incident involving a friend who received treatment for breast cancer. Her surgery had been uneventful. She went for the first round of chemotherapy with a sense of optimism, not knowing what to expect. There had been no discussion about how taxotere, carboplatin and herceptin (TCH) medication would work on the body, what the side-effects were or how to combat them. She was fine till the third day after treatment, when fatigue surfaced along with a profound nausea. Being absolutely unprepared, she handled it poorly. She took to bed, unable to consume much food or water. She developed day and night reversal, depression and dehydration. This led to a high-grade fever and urinary tract infection and required hospitalization.

Proper Counselling

Proper counselling of the patient and caregiver prior to chemotherapy, with an emphasis on proper hydration and diet to overcome the expected problems could have avoided the complications my friend had faced. Chemotherapy is toxic. A little help and guidance before treatment helps patients successfully navigate these difficulties, reducing complications and improving compliance. This experience had left her defeated. She wanted to stop treatment. Her oncologist suggested administration of only two drugs: carboplatin and herceptin (CH), eliminating taxotere, the most effective and potent drug, to reduce her toxicity. Her daughter and caregiver was greatly distressed, wanting more clarity on the further line of treatment.

There is no question that three drugs are better than two. They would have ensured maximum effect of treatment for her disease. The difficult period had been day three to six post the first round of chemotherapy. She needed a plan to keep herself **well hydrated, and nourished with multiple small meals and plenty of fluids, including green tea, coconut water and soups** for round two of chemotherapy. As the patient was an artist, she was advised to paint to occupy her time, along with listening to music or getting involved in any activity that interested her and could act as a diversion. With this advice, both physical and mental, she fared better during the second cycle of treatment and went on to complete all the cycles of chemotherapy.

The Body's Reaction to Chemotherapy

The traditional chemotherapeutic agents are cytotoxic. They act by killing cells that multiply rapidly—a characteristic of most malignant tumours. However, some normal cells in the body fall into this category too, particularly those of the gastro-intestinal system, bone marrow and hair follicles. This pool of normal rapidly dividing cells have to meet the body's demands during normal wear and tear, and they are also affected by the chemotherapeutic drugs.

Chemotherapy is stressful for the body. When highly potent and toxic drugs are injected directly into the bloodstream to suppress tumour growth, innocent bystander cells also take a hit. Maintaining a strong immune system reduces the risk of infection and improves the ability of the body to destroy surviving cancer cells. The food we eat must provide for all the body's demands during the illness, treatment and during the repair of the tissues. This is the diet-centric part of the therapy for cancer.

Importance of Good Nutrition

It is fundamental to recognize the importance of good nutrition during cancer therapy. The sum and substance of the diet is not only to provide nourishment—adequate intake of calories and other nutrients that the patient may require for the physical demands of the illness and the rigours of treatment—but also to maintain a steady weight to facilitate chemotherapy (since the dose of the drug is calculated according to the surface area or the weight of the patient) and to include foods with known anti-cancer effects.

Combating Gastro-Intestinal Side-Effects

The most common side-effects of chemotherapy are nausea, vomiting, anorexia, abdominal cramps, change in bowel habits, change in taste and smell, dental and gum problems and soreness of mouth depending on the type, dose, frequency and duration of treatment. These side-effects are not universal. When severe, they may lead to dehydration and malnutrition, especially when sustained over long periods of time. However, most of the symptoms last for three to four days after therapy, after which food is better tolerated.

The discharge summary given at the time of the completion of chemotherapy comes in handy. It often gives tips to overcoming common symptoms, remedies for vomiting and advice on bowel care. Generally, the side-effects are similar for subsequent cycles, although the severity may vary. Mostly, these are short-lived and require little treatment.

Some general precautions at home can reduce common side-effects. Kitchen or food smells that may trigger anorexia and nausea should be avoided. Eating multiple small meals keeps symptoms in check and ensures proper calorie intake. A change in taste can be achieved by frequent mouth washes with a **baking soda rinse**. Rinsing the mouth before and after each meal helps improve the taste. Drinking plenty of water and adding a slice of lime for variation in taste ensures adequate hydration.

> **Baking soda rinse:**
> 1 teaspoon of baking soda, 1 teaspoon of common salt in 1 litre of water. Mix well and keep the rinse at room temperature.

To overcome parosmia (altered smell), serve freshly cooked food at room temperature. Once the food cools, food smells reduce, making it easier to consume. Souring agents in the food like lime, lemon or vinegar improve flavour and reduce food smell. However, these additions may be troublesome when there are mouth ulcers. Black salt can be used as a substitute. **Lemon rice, curd rice, fish curries**, and **mango dal** all work well.[68] Eating frequent small meals, and drinking **ginger tea, green tea** or **buttermilk** between meals provides much-needed fluids for hydration and the removal of toxic waste from the body.

Mouth, Gum and Dental Side-Effects

Dental and gum problems may occur during chemotherapy. It is prudent to get a dental check-up and attend to all dental work before the start of chemotherapy. A sore mouth following treatment with chemotherapy or radiotherapy is the consequence of the treatment on the rapidly dividing cells of the mucous membrane of the mouth. Subsequent secondary infection occurs because of low immunity. The ulceration makes eating and swallowing difficult and often lasts for a few days.

- Management of mouth sores requires frequent mouth rinsing with the baking powder rinse, keeping mouth and teeth clean, using dental floss or Water Pik to clean between teeth, brushing teeth using a soft brush, and avoiding dentures if they cause discomfort.

- Application of vitamin E gently with a swab on the sore (puncture a 400 IU capsule of vitamin E and apply) promotes healing.
- Maintain good nutrition with a soft diet high in proteins.
- Avoid spicy food, and alcohol-containing mouthwashes, very hot or cold drinks, and citrus fruits for as long as the soreness remains.

Side-Effects on the Bone Marrow

The bone marrow contains precursor cells to all three elements of the blood—red blood cells, white blood cells and platelets. The precursor cells are all part of the normal pool of rapidly multiplying cells of the body, and are therefore targeted by chemotherapy. The effects can be **anaemia**, due to destruction of the red blood cells, resulting in insufficient oxygenation of the tissues; reduction in the white blood cells which predisposes the patient to **infections;** and **spontaneous bleeding** from the mucosa of the mouth and/or nose, due to the suppression of the platelets. When the reduction of any of these three elements is severe enough, it may delay further treatment and necessitate transfusions to correct the deficiency that has arisen.

An anecdotal report verbally communicated to me by a treating oncologist makes for interesting reading. Dr A. was treating a patient for cancer with multiple metastases, who required repeated platelet transfusions with each cycle of chemotherapy. Astonishingly, when the patient came in for his fourth cycle of treatment, the platelet count, which should have fallen significantly as on previous occasions, was reasonable and he did not require transfusion. When questioned, the patient revealed that his local doctor had suggested 'giloy' capsules to improve his count. He had taken these for three weeks, resulting in this improvement. He continued taking giloy, not requiring any further transfusions throughout the remainder of his chemotherapy. Giloy is a vine—also called *Tinospora cordifolia*, Indian Tinospora, or Gaduchi—which is widely used in Ayurveda, considered to be an immunity modulator and increases platelet counts. If the oncologist is agreeable, it may be tried.

Effect on Skin and Hair Follicles

Hair loss or alopecia is a temporary phenomenon. It may be accompanied by dry skin and brittle nails. The cells of the hair follicles are rapidly dividing and are therefore destroyed by chemotherapy. Hair loss can be severe. It requires no treatment. Eventually, a month or two after stoppage of treatment, the hair begins to sprout again and most of it grows back over a period of time.

Miscellaneous Effects: Cancer Fatigue

Fatigue may be a consequence of the cancer treatment, be it chemotherapy or radiation. It is unpredictable, yet it is one of the most distressing side-effects. It is often worse immediately after the treatment, persisting for a few days before reducing slowly in time for the next cycle. The level of fatigue may increase as treatment continues. Many factors compound the fatigue: low levels of red blood cells, sleeping problems, loss of appetite resulting in poor nutrition and lack of exercise.

I am reminded of my friend Anil, who had developed progressive Stage IV colon cancer. His oncologist had suggested a trial of three cycles of chemotherapy, including a drug that blocked new blood vessel formation. I visited him on the tenth day of his first cycle. He had severe fatigue, barely managing to sit up for two minutes to sip water.

His voice was faint. He was struggling to eat. He was most comfortable lying in a foetal position.

After a discussion on the causes for his fatigue that so overwhelmed him, we deduced that it was the progression of his cancer, the effects of chemotherapy and the lack of nourishment. In addition to the antidepressant the oncologist had prescribed, it was suggested that some of his needs could be met by consuming six to eight small meals, which included foods rich in protein, vitamins and minerals. He promised to make an attempt to improve his diet after realizing that the hollow feeling in the abdomen was hunger, and not the cancer growing rapidly. Ten days later I met him again—he had decided to stop further chemotherapy and was on multiple small meals daily. He felt better for it. His voice was stronger, he could sit up, and he even walked to the table for lunch.

Other reasons for fatigue are increased energy requirement for repair and healing of damaged tissues, build-up of toxic substances from cell destruction due to the treatment, and the challenges faced by the immune system during treatment. Adequate fluid intake and exercise are ways to flush out the accumulated toxins.

Management of Cancer Fatigue

Fatigue is a side-effect that needs proper handling and management. Some of the causes are food-related and can be factored into the diet—like eating foods rich in proteins, vitamins and minerals, or protein supplements and vitamin tablets to deal with anaemia, along with extra proteins for tissue repair.

Apart from food, many other factors can help in alleviating fatigue:

- Building a new routine created by the patient can ensure better time management. They should undertake some exercise like short walks, listen to music, read—whatever is of interest to the individual. These help patients remain focused, preventing day-night reversal, reduce stress, and promote relaxation by participating in activities that are light and meaningful. Involvement in day-to-day activities at home or work helps to keep depression at bay.

- When fatigue is profound immediately after chemotherapy, short rest-breaks, three to four times a day, balanced with some activity, are ideal.
- Avoid long rest-breaks or sleeping all day. Conversely, although it is important for patients to remain active, they should not be pushed excessively.
- Daily exercise improves appetite and prevents constipation.
- Sunning oneself helps relax the body, elevates the mood and provides the much-needed daily supply of Vitamin D.

FOODS TO BOOST THE IMMUNE SYSTEM

- Vitamins, proteins and omega-3 must be provided in the diet.
- Vegetables that can be washed well, preferably soaked and scrubbed, should be eaten. The food-preparing counter must be cleaned before and after each use.
- Eat fruits that can be peeled, i.e. avoiding the peels of fruits like pears, peaches and apples, etc.
- Tomatoes should be soaked in boiling water before adding to the salad.
- Microwave meat and chicken for rapid thawing and then cook immediately.
- Anaemia requires foods rich in iron, folic acid and B12 (see p. 98 in 'Surgery and Nutrition').

Foods to Be Avoided

Food safety becomes a priority during treatment. Both chemotherapy and radiotherapy weaken the immune system. Diarrhoea can be problematic. During treatment avoid raw vegetables like sprouts, lettuce, frozen foods, smoked fish and pate, sushi and sashimi, raw milk or cheeses made from un-pasteurized milk, uncooked eggs, non-homemade salads and sandwiches. Eat only freshly cooked food, not leftovers, reheated or frozen and thawed food.

On one occasion, I met a friend just before his first dose of chemotherapy. He had had surgery for cancer of the colon. It was lunchtime, and he was getting admitted that afternoon for chemotherapy. He was calm; it was his first cycle. I was taken aback with what he ate for lunch: a slice of thick-crust pizza that was left over from a previous meal. It had been frozen and was thawed that morning for him. There was also a salad where most of the greens were raw, along with a bowl of yogurt.

Even at the best of times, fast foods must to be avoided. But stale food, even though frozen, spells big trouble. That friend developed diarrhoea during chemotherapy. Was the diarrhoea only due to chemotherapy, or had the stale frozen pizza contributed to it? I cannot say, but I must emphasize again the need to eat freshly cooked, light food before chemotherapy.

Food Time-table for Chemotherapy

Whichever meal works well should be eaten to the fullest. **Breakfast** is the meal that is generally best tolerated.

7:30 a.m.: Freshly made mixed fruit juice (See p. 97).

8 a.m.: Sugar-free cereal with flax seeds and cinnamon/ upma/egg and toast with tea. Boiled or scrambled eggs, one to two whole grain toasts OR hot or cold cereal are easy to consume.

11:30 a.m.: Yogurt with 1 tablespoon of mixed nuts. Yogurt with berries also works well, and can be eaten between meals.

1:30 p.m.: Soft food—khichri cooked with vegetables, dal and rice. Chopped chicken can be added if desired.

4:30 p.m: Stewed fruits and a cup of tea. Bananas are a good snack.

6 p.m.: Soup (See p. 122–23 in 'Managing Palliative Care').

8 p.m.: Dinner—similar to lunch. Cup of green tea after dinner.

Radiation Therapy and Nutrition

Cure sometimes, treat often, comfort always.

—Hippocrates

Radiation therapy, like chemotherapy, kills rapidly dividing cancer cells. But additionally, it also affects rapidly dividing normal tissue in the vicinity of the tumour. The cells most affected are in the S and M phase of the cell cycle (see p. 32 in 'Cancer Treatments').

The damage to normal cells causes unwanted side-effects. This treatment, therefore, involves maintaining a balance between destroying the cancer cells and minimizing the effects on normal tissue. Unlike chemotherapy, the cell destruction by radiation does not necessarily occur right away. At times, it may take days or weeks after the exposure to radiation for the cells to self-destruct. Normal tissues, made up of rapidly growing cells like skin and bone marrow, are often affected earlier than the tumour. Others tissues like nerves, brain and breast generally show late effects. It is for this reason that this form of treatment may still cause side-effects long after the therapy is over.

Side-Effects of Radiation Therapy

Advances in radiation therapy, like Image-Guided Radiation, accurately focus the radiation on to the diseased tissue. While this minimizes the side-effects, some fibrosis of normal tissue may still occur. Since the treatment is localized, the side-effects depend on the area of the body receiving the treatment.

Common side-effects are: fatigue, skin changes, lymphoedema, low blood counts, loss of appetite, nausea, vomiting, diarrhoea and secondary tumours.

Fatigue

The extreme tiredness that follows radiation not relieved by rest is often labelled as fatigue. There is no single cause for fatigue, nor any single treatment for it (see p 107–09 in 'Chemotherapy and Nutrition').

Skin Changes

Faint redness of the skin surface may develop and progress to tenderness, blistering, and dryness. Peeling of skin mostly occurs three to four weeks after the start of treatment. It resembles a case of severe sunburn. Hair loss over the treated area is common. Moisturizing the skin or taking Vitamin E supplements may help once treatment is over.

During the period of treatment avoid the following: exposure to the sun (the skin is sensitive to sunlight), moisturizers, soap, deodorant or perfume. Avoid scrubbing the area or applying hot or cold packs. Wear loose, soft garments to allow for proper blood circulation.

Lymphoedema

The blockage of the lymphatic vessels causing swelling of the limb that results from the accumulation of body fluid in the tissue is called lymphoedema. The lymph nodes in the axilla are removed during surgery for breast cancer. These lymph nodes not only drain the breast tissue but also the entire arm. Their removal is necessary to prevent the spread of the disease via the lymphatic vessels and also for staging the cancer. Radiation therapy given for breast cancer not only targets the breast, but also the axilla. This may result in the blockage of the lymphatic vessels, in an already compromised lymphatic system (since the lymph nodes have been surgically removed). The blockage of the lymphatic vessels interferes with the drainage of the lymph fluid (interstitial or body fluids) from the arm, resulting in its collection in the soft tissue and the development of lymphoedema of the affected arm. After radiation ends, this side-effect lasts for three to four weeks, but at times may persist for longer.

Secondary Tumours

The risk of secondary tumours developing in the same location, or in nearby organs, has been reported after radiation therapy. Though the incidence is small in number, these are a cause for concern.

I recall reporting on the biopsy of eighty-seven-year-old Mrs G. She developed cancer of the left cheek, but was a non-smoker and did not chew tobacco or eat betel nut. After careful questioning, she revealed having had treatment for breast cancer on the left side twenty-five years ago—this had included radiation therapy. Those were the days of less precise radiation. Her tumour in the cheek was likely a secondary cancer occurring post-radiation therapy. Fortunately, the focused radiation technique has significantly reduced this side-effect.

Miscellaneous Effects

Head and neck radiation may cause dryness of mouth, loss of taste, and thick, rope-like saliva. These side-effects are short-lived and disappear over time. If problems persist consult the oncologist.

Nausea, vomiting and headaches may be delayed side-effects of radiation to the head and neck region. Nutrition should not be the casualty during treatment (for the management of the symptoms, refer to p. 104–05 in 'Chemotherapy and Nutrition').

DIET DURING RADIATION THERAPY

- The body needs adequate calories, proteins and vitamins for its energy demands, repair and healing (as given for surgery)—during and after radiation therapy.
- It is important not to lose weight during treatment as the radiation therapy plan is specific to the patients' size and shape.
- When appetite is a problem, extra energy and proteins can be added to the diet without having to actually consume extra food (see p. xx in 'Managing Palliative Care').
- High energy drinks like milkshakes or soup (see p. 122-23) work well.
- Hydration, by consuming plenty of fluids including water and tea, is important for healing.
- Have many small meals rather than large meals; six to eight small meals instead of three full meals will take care of the calorie requirements.
- Have a soft or a liquid diet if swallowing is a problem.
- Avoid alcohol or spicy food in case of mouth ulcers.
- Energy foods and proteins form the backbone of the diet during radiotherapy.
- Food safety (see p. 110) should be carefully adhered to, ensuring that the food is cooked at proper temperature and avoiding raw foods.
- If diarrhoea develops after lower abdominal radiation, probiotics like yogurt can be eaten.

Managing Palliative Care

It is not how long you live, but how well you do it.

—Martin Luther King Jr.

Depending on the type of primary tumour, a cancer may progress by local recurrence or spread to distant sites, often involving the lymph node and vital organs like the liver, lungs, kidneys and brain. This distant spread is known as metastasis.

When all forms of treatments, be it surgery, or various combinations of chemotherapy or radiotherapy, have failed to curtail the disease and the cancer continues to spreads unchecked, it is known as cancer progression. Any type of therapy given to the patient from this point onwards is unlikely to benefit them, since the cancer has been found to be resistant to treatment. Whatever treatment is given may cause extreme toxicity and therefore a great deal of discomfort. When toxicity outweighs the benefits, when the side-effects cause more harm to the patient than the disease per se, and the quality of life suffers, what is the answer then?

All treatments targeting the cancer are withdrawn, and the patient moves to supportive or palliative care. Here one falls back on symptomatic care and a diet to maintain the nutritional needs of the patient.

Palliative Care, Pain and Nutrition

Palliative care is a multidisciplinary approach designed to improve the quality of life in serious, life-limiting illnesses like cancer that are beyond cure. It focuses on providing supportive care to relieve symptoms like pain, depression, breathlessness, fatigue, insomnia, loss of appetite as well as spiritual problems that may arise.

Patients are generally unaware of what to expect at the end of life. They need guidance, and also the *whole truth* regarding the condition of their health. Understanding the complete picture enables them to make informed decisions. Every coordinate must be known before embarking on this end-of-life voyage. The solace provided helps the patient live their lives as completely and comfortably as possible.

One view suggests that palliative care should actually begin at the time of the diagnosis of cancer and continue throughout treatment, with follow-up care and end-of-life support towards the end. Instituting early palliative care was recommended in 1990 by the World Health Organization.[69] Towards the end of 1990, based on two studies on end-of-life care, an expert panel documented the problems of patients and their needs.[70] These centred around communication between the doctor, the family and the caregiver, addressing emotional issues and depression, as well as fulfilling the spiritual needs of the patient.

The Need for Palliative Care

The team for palliative care should ideally comprise a doctor, a nurse, a social worker/counsellor and a priest. Such a team would be geared not only to give solace to the patient, but also to help provide extra support and guidance to the care-givers and other family members that may help them deal with any kind of eventuality. Once contact and trust have been established, periodic visits or discussions with such a team would mitigate problems like pain, improving food intake and dealing with depression when they arise. This kind of care can be provided wherever desired, be it at home, in a hospital or a hospice.

In India, a caregiver is normally a family member—spouse, parent, son, daughter, or a sibling, sometimes even a friend—who helps the individual with the activities of daily living. The impact of having a terminally-ill patient at home on the family is profound. In such a predicament, it is necessary to include all members of the family, even children, and keep them abreast of the situation. Understanding the gravity of the illness through discussion not only provides involvement, but also the strength to endure the outcome of the illness. Moreover, it prevents anxiety and depression from setting in, which benefits everyone.

I met a friend whose son developed problems as a result of inadequate involvement in his father's care. They were a family of four and the father was diagnosed with terminal lung cancer. The mother was the primary caregiver. The daughter was in her late teens and had assisted her mother whenever the need arose. The son, in his early teens, was unaware of the seriousness of the situation. In fact, because of his age, family and friends were overprotective and shielded him from the reality.

The father died three months after being diagnosed and the young teenager was confused and consumed with guilt at not having done enough for his father. He failed in his final exam. It took him the better part of two years and multiple visits to a counsellor to overcome his guilt. People say that *death is fulfillment of life*, yet a death in the family had left this boy bereft and shattered, with little comprehension of why his life had changed so completely. Including him in the discussion earlier and involving him in the care of his father may have helped him understand and ultimately, cope better with the situation.

Palliative care touches on all aspects of a person's life and illness. Problems that arise are addressed as soon as they appear. As a result, the patient feels better cared for at all times, and the caregiver gets the appropriate and necessary guidance. Studies conducted on patients with metastatic cancer have suggested a significantly better outcome, in relation to the quality of life, mood and long-time survival, when palliative care was started early on in the course of treatment.[71] This holistic approach to treatment, going beyond treating the disease, is enormously comforting to the patient and the family. Even caregivers of the patients receiving early palliative care fared better and had lower rates of depression.[72]

Due to the numerous demands of the illness on the body, the recommendations for healthy eating differ from that of normal individuals. Before addressing nutritional concerns, it is essential to assist with any physical symptoms such as pain and sleeping trouble. It is also important to recognize and find solutions to social, mental and spiritual problems. Loss of appetite and nausea need attention too—their management has been detailed earlier in this book, (see p. 104–05). Once all these problems are ameliorated, it is easier to concentrate on nourishment.

Managing Pain

The threshold and tolerance for pain varies from person to person. However, once pain appears, however mild it may be, it needs immediate attention and management, and it should not be ignored. A record of the levels of pain, on a scale of 10, could be maintained by the patient before pain therapy is started. This measurement can be used as a yardstick for further pain management. Any variation in the pain, whether in the day or at night, should also be noted.

The best approach to pain care is the preventive approach: start treatment early when the symptoms are mild. If suffering is controlled, it automatically improves the quality of life. The patient eats better, sleeps well and the mood remains uplifted.

Great inroads have been made in the understanding of pain therapy. It is possible to keep the patient pain-free at all times with round-the-clock medication. Dosage adjustments are made whenever pain reappears. Stronger medication can be introduced when needed. Many drug combinations work their magic through the different pain pathways, each tackled individually. The WHO ladder for cancer pain is an inexpensive and effective method for relieving cancer pain in up to 90 per cent of patients.[73]

Managing Sleep

Apart from pain, there are many causes of sleeping disorders in patients with cancer. Attempts could be made to reduce dependence on sleep medication. One should use either natural or artificial lamps to provide light stimulation therapy. Timed light exposure helps regulate the circadian rhythm and establish a regular sleep-wake cycle. The circadian rhythm is a twenty-four-hour cycle of physical, mental and behavioural changes that are common to most living things and occur in response to light and darkness.

Other measures that also help are:

- Deep breathing exercises for relaxation;
- Maintaining sleep hygiene by going to bed more or less at the same time daily;
- Not trying to sleep immediately after a heavy meal;
- Stimulus control by spending less time lying down in bed;
- Stress reduction;
- Sleep restriction procedures to limit day-time sleeping.

Managing the Daily Routine

Providing a routine to the patient, with many activities such as meeting friends and other social interactions, exercise, regular meals, and recreational activities and hobbies, gives some structure to the patient's day. These need to be factored into the time-table.

Managing Nutrition

Even though it may be short-lived, the immediate effect of the withdrawal of chemotherapy is the improvement in the patient's general condition. Gradually, some of the toxic effects of the treatment begin to fade away. The relief, after the long arduous journey through unrelenting chemotherapy, often with complications, is dramatic and welcome. The appetite improves, nausea and fatigue decrease. The need of the hour is to capitalize on this situation and provide all the nutritional support possible. Food acts as a survivorship intervention—its major goal is to minimize cachexia.

Cachexia

In palliative care, the main focus of nutrition is on improving the quality of life and relieving suffering. Cachexia is a wasting syndrome with extreme, progressive and persistent weight loss. It occurs in many chronic diseases as well as in cancer. It is caused by a large group of substances called cytokines. These may be proteins, peptides, or glycoproteins that are secreted by specific cells of the immune system to mediate and regulate immunity, inflammation and white blood cell formation. They are produced as a natural defence against malignancy or inflammation. However, the immunological overreach, meant to alleviate inflammation, comes back to haunt the body. These substances act as double-edged swords—initially, as helpful molecules fighting the disease; however, their overproduction for sustained periods of time can act as a signal for cachexia.

To maximize health benefits and to get the best results, nutritional changes should be introduced early in the course of the disease. The philosophy here is to make every gulp and morsel count. Increasing the frequency of meals from six to eight per day may be the answer. Calories and proteins should be ensured with every meal or snack (owing to the decreased appetite of the patient). This may entail the use of nutrients like fish oil, vitamins and selective nutritional supplements of proteins.

Proteins are the building blocks for the repair and

maintenance of muscle mass, as well as a necessity for propping up the immune system. The protein needs of patients may be double that of normal individuals. The usual everyday requirement is 0.8 grams of protein per kilogram of body weight per day. This should be increased to 1.4 to 2 grams per kilogram of body weight per day.

RECOMMENDATIONS FOR INCREASING PROTEIN INTAKE

- Fortified milk: Add one cup of skimmed milk powder to 1 litre of full cream milk or 1 cup of evaporated milk to 2 cups of regular milk. This milk should be used for the patient's every need, including cereal, coffee, milk drink with chocolate, milkshake with banana, or even to set yogurt.
- Add protein powder to fruit or vegetable juice.
- Nutritional supplements such as commercial protein powders with minerals and vitamins should be used. These can be mixed in milk to provide extra proteins.
- The patient can be fed every two hours when the intake of food is markedly reduced. To help with compliance, the day's menu should be discussed with the patient.

A Meal In a Bowl

Soups can serve as a complete meal. A soup is easy to consume and can provide for most of the nutritional needs of the patients, particularly when the loss of appetite is severe. The stock gives body to the soup and provides much-needed proteins. The stock can be made from chicken, meat or lentils, depending on the preferences of the patients.

<u>Meat/Chicken Stock (5 servings):</u>

1. Wash ½ kg mutton bones with some meat on them well. A couple of marrow bones in addition give

better flavour. For chicken stock, use half a medium chicken with bones in place of the mutton bones.

2. Add meat, bones and sufficient water, about 2 to 2½ litres and bring to a rolling boil.
3. Turn down to a simmer and skim any foam that collects.
4. Now add 1 teaspoon salt, ¼ medium sliced onions, 2 bay leaves, ½ small chopped turnip, a sprig of parsley and 4 to 6 peppercorns.
5. Simmer partially covered for one and a half hours. This ensures the maximum extraction from the meat.
6. Strain through two layers of coarse cloth.
7. Cool, skim off fat that forms a crust on top.
8. If greater concentration is required, simmer further to desired taste.

Lentil Stock (5 servings):

1. Wash 1 cup lentils.
2. Boil in 6 cups of water. Bring to a rolling boil.
3. Turn down to a simmer add 1 teaspoon salt, 1 small onion sliced, 1 bay leaf, ½ turnip chopped, 4-6 peppercorns, ½ teaspoon each of turmeric, cumin and coriander seed powder.
4. Simmer for half an hour. Skim off the froth.
5. Pass through a sieve.

Note:

After preparing the stock using the above recipes, one can make all kinds of soups: lentil, mixed vegetable, cream of tomato/carrot/broccoli/mushroom, pumpkin or fish soup.

Part III

A JOURNEY WITH CANCER

Diagnosis and Starting Treatment

Health is not valued till sickness comes.

—Thomas Fuller

Arun had just celebrated his sixty-second birthday. He was content and happy with how life had panned out for him. His first grandchild was due in early July, something he had always looked forward to, since he loved little children. These were exciting times.

On the night of 11 May, 2010, he said, 'The rheumatism from my childhood has returned; only this time it is not in the knees but in my left hip.' I gave him a pain-killer that night, and he slept. Prior to this, he had had no symptoms—neither pain, nor urinary retention.

The next day we had an appointment with the orthopaedic surgeon at four in the afternoon. The doctor examined him and ordered blood tests and x-rays of the left hip and pelvis. The blood tests revealed elevated Prostate-Specific Antigens (PSA). The remaining blood profile was normal. The x-ray failed to show any significant abnormality. His last PSA, done in May 2007, had been within the normal range. He had slipped up on getting his routine check-up as our son was getting married towards the end of 2008.

At the time he had said, 'I have too much on my plate. All my previous tests were normal. I feel fine. I have no symptoms, let me be.'

An elevated PSA in itself is not enough for a diagnosis of prostate cancer. Further investigations and a visit to the urologist were necessary. A digital rectal examination, ultrasound of the lower abdomen to assess the size of the prostate, and bone scans were required. The confirmatory test would be a prostate biopsy.

We went to the urologist in a new facility in Gurugram.

He advised a prostate biopsy. Four days later, we had a report of prostate cancer, Gleason score 7. Though twelve cores were taken, representative tissue was present in only three. Meanwhile, the ultrasound and bone scan concluded: 'Cancer prostate with multiple bone metastasis and locally advanced disease involving the seminal vesicles'. An MRI test was now obligatory to rule out compression of the spinal nerves by the growing cancer. Fortunately, the pain was not due to pressure on the nerves.

For Arun, the disease had already spread beyond the prostate, so surgery was not an option. There was no compression of the spinal nerves, therefore no radiotherapy was required. Arun needed a medical oncologist to start treatment, preferably one who inspired confidence. Someone he was willing to trust because of his knowledge, his humility and his compassion. We went to Dr AA, a senior oncologist with good communication skills. Interestingly, we only met an oncologist—there was no team involved, not even a dietician.

Arun had a forty-five minute discussion with the oncologist regarding his treatment and the likely outcome. He used all his journalistic skills to question the doctor and get the answers he was looking for. 'I can treat your disease, but I cannot cure you,' the doctor said at the outset.

Arun asked, 'How many years do you give me and what will be the quality of my life?'

'If all goes well, you have about seven to ten years, but it depends on your response to the treatment. I will start with androgen deprivation therapy (ADT). Prostate cancer thrives on androgens—blocking the hormone will result in shrinkage of the tumour, the immediate effect of which will be the disappearance of pain. The growth and spread of the disease will be suppressed. However, the tumour will not melt away. I will only switch to chemotherapy once the disease becomes resistant to ADT. The quality of life will be as before.'

This discussion with the oncologist was reassuring and Arun felt comfortable about his prospects. He was willing to go ahead with the treatment. He was started on two anti-androgens (Casodex and Zoladex). Zoledronic acid was given to strengthen the bone and prevent bone breakdown or fractures due to the metastasis. Zoledronic acid and Zoladex would be administered throughout his years of treatment, irrespective of whether he received ADT or chemotherapy.

Ten days after his presenting symptom of pain began, ADT was started. A week later, he was completely pain-free. The disappearance of pain, as expected, greatly increased Arun's faith in the doctor, lowered his stress levels, and restored his belief in himself. He felt he had the wherewithal to fight the cancer.

During the period between the onset of pain and the start of treatment, Arun had not stopped working, even though the pain put paid to his morning walks. As soon as he was pain-free, he felt confident enough to restart his walks. Life had a purpose again. He was back to meeting friends and enjoying his food. A month later, he was ready to travel again. Arun had no side-effects from this treatment and began to eat a diet specially modified for him, with the addition of green tea, wheatgrass juice and a salad before every meal.

Travelling Again

To travel is to take a journey into yourself.

—Danny Kaye

Until before his cancer diagnosis, Arun was fond of three things: food, travel, and the company of friends. They had been the essence of his very being, and for him they determined his quality of life. A month after the start of his treatment, since there were no restrictions on food and travel, we went to Kashmir for fifteen days. We spent seven days in Srinagar at a boutique hotel on the Nagin lake, before going on to Gulmarg. In Srinagar, the Kashmiri wazwan was delightful and made up for the restriction in movement due to a lockdown. Things appeared to be steadily getting better and back on track for Arun. Gulmarg, too, worked out well. I was pleased to see Arun navigate the slopes without much difficulty. It was paramount, given the situation, to maintain normalcy as far as possible.

On the morning of the last day of our trip we got the good news about our grandson's arrival. Babies have a tendency to take you by surprise—he was born a week before the due date. The excitement was palpable. On our journey down from Gulmarg to Srinagar, we seemed to be flying. Arun put his weight behind the car to propel us faster.

We arrived in Delhi by three in the afternoon. I suspect Arun was a bit tired, but we went straight from the airport to the hospital to see the mother and child. Arman, the new entrant into our family, soon became his only love. Arman was the most beautiful thing that had happened to him. He said, 'Just holding him is soothing to my soul. It has made everything in life worthwhile.' He now had a new purpose to his life.

Three months after his treatment had started, Arun's

PSA was below one. Radiological findings showed that some of his bone lesions had regressed, while others had cleared completely. Happy with this outcome, he wanted to try a longer journey in August. We went to Switzerland, the country he considered the most civilized and decent. He had worked and lived there for seven years in his fifties.

He knew his time was limited, and he was feeling better. Besides, travel was a passion and he had to be on the move. It was summer and Switzerland was at its most picturesque, with flowers growing along the pavements, colour-coordinated and landscaped. Everything was exceedingly clean. Despite there being many more people in the towns and villages, and many more houses than a decade earlier, it was still like a picture-perfect postcard in whichever direction we looked. We stayed in the French part of the country, travelling to familiar haunts and eating some delectable French food. The time spent in Switzerland was never enough for Arun.

We went on to Belgium to spend three days in a charming, small and old pre-Roman town with a Dutch influence called Bruges. It had old, narrow cobblestone streets, many canals and waterways, and excellent chocolate, beer and food. The street food, like waffles with strawberries and cream, was superb. The town itself had no transport except at a few places and we walked, seeking out the many recommended restaurants. Arun never tired when there was good food on the other side.

At the best of times, Arun had been a great planner and the best guide on any travel. He extensively researched a place—its cuisine, historic sites, almost anything you could think of—and it was all done well before any trip. His study was so complete that it felt as if he had been there before.

That December, after Christmas, we went to Pondicherry as a family—three different generations. It was an exceptional trip, and he got to spend quality time with his grandson. To top it all, there was interesting French and Vietnamese food on offer.

Arun's condition remained stable and he managed to do all the things that were crucial for his well-being. His quality of life was good for the time being. There was complete physical, mental and social well-being. There were no gaps, at this point, between his hopes and expectations, and his present experiences. He was at peace with himself. Come what may, he visited his grandson Arman daily.

In May 2011, we travelled to China. Shanghai was a spanking new city, yet it was a place without a soul. We could have been anywhere in the world—there was nothing Chinese about this city, except the people. The historical pottery collection on display at the museum was the personal acquisition of a baron from Hong Kong. The French and British influences were apparent but old Chinese Shanghai was difficult to find.

There were no children in the streets or in the shops. There were no elderly people either. We must have been the oldest couple there. The entire population of the city seemed to range between 20-40 years, and everyone was in an enormous hurry. We wanted to buy a security blanket for Arman, our grandson, and it was only on the evening of the third day of our trip, after much searching, that we discovered a small children's store in a mall. Without any more shopping to worry about, we could finally enjoy our trip.

We did all the touristy things, seeing the terracotta warriors and the Big Wild Goose Pagoda in Xian. We even ate a meal of what tasted like keema paratha in the Muslim quarter, wondering if Hiuen Tsang had, along with the Buddhist scriptures, brought the parathas back to China from India. The best food, of course, was in Beijing. It was different from Indian-Chinese food but quite delicious. We stuck to seafood, chicken and duck, never quite sure what the other meats were. Fifteen days later, having visited the Great Wall of China, Tiananmen Square, and the Forbidden City, we happily returned to Delhi with Arman's blanket.

The China trip did wonders for Arun's confidence. He was now ready to do short trips on his own. He made multiple trips to Goa, Kerala, Bangalore and Lucknow, some of which were work-related while others were for pleasure. We even managed a short road trip to Simla, staying at a bed-and-breakfast called 'Sunny Mead' with my niece, and having the most exceptional home-cooked food. The first seven months of 2011 went by like a breeze, without a hitch. Three monthly blood tests and radiology reassured us that the disease was currently in check. He was in partial remission.

Maintaining Nutrition While Travelling

Culinary experience is an integral part of the pleasures of travel. However, travel can be disruptive on the diet, particularly while on medication. By following the broad outlines given for a healthy diet (see p. 67–68 in 'The Relationship Between Cancer and Food'), these challenges can be overcome and imbalances can be prevented, particularly while on a long cruise or trip.

In Srinagar, the Kashmiri food where we stayed was largely non-vegetarian, centred around lamb/mutton, which is often cooked with yogurt, using little or no onions or garlic. Ordinarily, on the menu there were always some curries with the meat cooked with vegetables (not potato). This could be eaten along with a saag (spinach) substituting for the salad.

There is wisdom in finishing a meal with a fruit rather than a dessert rich in refined carbohydrates and sugar. This is true for the Western diet as well, which should ideally start with a salad in vinegar-oil dressing, then a main course of chicken or fish, and avoiding the heavy desserts. For Chinese food, including sautéed vegetables or a salad works well in the meal. While travelling, the menu at every meal requires careful study, selecting dishes that ensure adequate fruits and vegetables. Foods satisfying not only the health requirement but also the taste should be eaten.

Dealing With Cancer

Though travelling was a complete distraction from the disease, anxiety did surface at times. Arun was not one to complain about the hand he had been dealt. He was stoic about his disease, generally keeping it out of his conversation, even from me. Was this his way of preventing the disease from affecting his spirits or was it a way of overcoming his anxiety for what lay ahead? Everyone reacts differently to a serious illness. As we cannot wish it away, it is better to face it head on. I have always felt that being better informed about the disease, participating actively in every aspect of the illness, and looking after your body and mind improves the harmony within you, and enhances your ability to heal. This complete involvement achieves mobilization of the body to fight the disease better. Putting a problem on the backburner is no solution. Arun read extensively about his disease but remained stoic, and did not encourage much discussion. This was his sanctuary in dealing with the situation he found himself in.

Change in Medication

There is nothing permanent except change.
—Heraclitus

So far all had gone well. During his monthly follow-up on the treatment strategy being followed by Arun, his oncologist had used three parameters to judge the success of the treatment and advancement of the disease, in order to decide when it was time to change medication. The parameters were: rising trend of PSA, reappearance of symptoms and unequivocal increase in the number of lesions from radiology. Though radiology alone was the single-most important criteria—the appearance of even a single new lesion was enough to start a new drug—if any two of the three parameters were positive on two consecutive consultations, the decision for change was apparent. In early September 2011, Arun's PSA was rising and some pain began to appear off and on.

Casodex—the anti-androgen drug—was stopped and Ketoconazole and Prednisone were started. Ketoconazole would inhibit testicular and adrenal steroid production, while Prednisone was replacement therapy—replacing the essential corticoids depleted by Ketoconazole. These corticoids, normally produced by the adrenals, were necessary for maintaining life. The toxicity encountered by Arun was followed by minimal nausea—short-lived and overcome by frequent mouth-washing and sugar-free mint. These were oral medicines—easy to administer and carry on trips—and Arun was comfortable taking them.

Alternative Remedies

Arun was a great believer in homeopathy, partly because of his childhood experiences with this form of medication. The homeopath gave him medication to boost his immune system.

'There is nothing specific for the cancer in homeopathy,' he said. Arun took the homeopathic pills simultaneously with the other drugs. These pills were of such miniscule doses that they were unlikely to produce any side-effects, or have any interplay with the other medications he was taking.

In the third week of September, our second grandchild, Seher, was born. As the radiologist had not revealed the gender of the child on ultrasound (not permitted by law) but had made similar pronouncements as for the first pregnancy, it was assumed that it would be another boy. There was much excitement when a girl child was born instead. It was the first girl to be born in Arun's family in three generations. Arun loved both his grandchildren dearly, but he always had a special bond with Arman. Possibly, it was because Arman was the first grandchild, but I suspect it was more because he looked just like Adil, our son, at that age. For Arun, it was like having his fully-grown son along with this child version of him, both at the same time.

At the beginning of December 2011, Arun had written about the progression of his disease and the fatigue he sometimes felt to his friend and cousin, George Verghese (known to us as Reji), a professor at MIT. Reji was very perceptive and connected Arun to Dr Paul Mathew, an oncologist in Boston with expertise in prostate cancer. Email communication with Paul was established. All details of previous treatment, blood tests and radiological investigations were sent. Dr Mathew had been greatly reassuring and had managed to placate Arun with the long list of alternative remedies available to him. Henceforth, all information regarding the progress of his disease and any regimen change were first vetted by Paul. He advised him on an exercise routine and a change in diet in order to overcome the fatigue he had recently developed.

Regular physical activity may have a protective role against cancer—tempering the adverse effects of treatment. It is true that patients experience fatigue during chemotherapy and radiation therapy but exercise has the opposite effect. It improves muscle power, cardio-respiratory function and quality of life. Improving the circulation provides more oxygen to the cells which, in itself, is detrimental to the cancer.

Another Change In Medication

After Christmas 2011, the monthly PSA had again started showing an upward trend. Though he had remained symptom-free, a CT scan showed a thickening of the bladder wall. The oncologist was of the opinion that the previous combination of drugs was no longer effective and replaced them with Honvan, another oral anti-androgen drug.

Honvan is a synthetic oestrogen that is converted to an active form in the body. It acts by lowering the levels of androgens, resulting in reduction of the size of the tumour. Arun continued to work and lead a normal life. He managed to visit his grandchildren as part of his daily routine, also meeting with friends and going on walks as before.

In the second week of January we went to Cochin for six days. Arun wanted his dose of Kerala food. For this, nothing was better than the food at The Grand Hotel, and we lunched there daily. The cuisine was authentic Syrian Christian—very fresh and quite delicious. In fact, the seafood comprised of that morning's catch. The fried prawns, meen pollichathu (fish in banana leaves), and coconut meat were the highlights. On the second day at lunch, as we awaited our food, a couple walked in. The man looked like a local, the woman was Caucasian, and with them was a little girl. They took the table adjacent to ours.

Suddenly, Arun got up from his chair and went up to the recently-arrived gentleman. I heard him say, 'Are you Dr Paul Mathew?' Paul was completely blown away. Here he was in Kerala, on holiday from Boston with his family, and an unknown person had recognized him. A month earlier, while emailing him, Arun had seen his photograph on the web. He never forgot a face and had easily identified him. Paul proved to be a friend, an understanding and caring oncologist, always factual, logical and down to earth, pushing us in the right direction.

Caring for Others

The character of a man is his guardian spirit.

—Unknown

Arun had family in Malaysia. These were much older cousins from Kerala who had moved there towards the end of the Second World War. Their children were his age, rather than the cousins themselves. Over the years, he had travelled on many occasions to Kuala Lumpur (KL) and Penang and met most of them. Typical of Indian immigrants, the second-generation had done exceedingly well, both educationally and socially. Most were doctors, dentists or lawyers, and even judges.

Visiting a Cousin with Cancer

In early March 2012, we received a call from Malaysia from a nephew of his afflicted with renal cell carcinoma. He was terminally ill, and had the desire to meet with Arun. We had been in touch for two decades and had met him on most of our previous visits. Recently, he had developed recurrent disease and multiple metastases. His health had declined over the last month and now he was having difficulty getting out of bed.

There is something you cannot help but notice about people who are suffering from a serious illness—their own vulnerability makes them more caring and compassionate about other people. With Arun it was the same. He immediately agreed to visit his nephew. The wishes of the dying should always be fulfilled.

Fifteen days later, we flew into Kuala Lumpur. The first night there was a family reunion, where more than twenty relatives came for dinner. It was an honour for Arun and he enjoyed the attention. It was a proud moment for him to see the success of his family in Malaysia, with each generation becoming more prosperous than the last.

The next evening we travelled to the outskirts of KL to meet with Arun's ailing nephew. Suresh's condition had not permitted him to attend the family dinner the previous evening. We got there at six in the evening and chatted with Suresh's wife, Shanta, for half an hour. Suresh was nowhere to be seen and Arun was getting impatient. Another fifteen minutes passed when suddenly a door opened and out walked Suresh. He was very unstable even with a walker, and deathly pale. But it looked like he had a second wind in his sails. He had managed to give it his all to walk out and meet us.

Where there is a will, there is a way.

He was overwhelmed to see us. 'Because of you,' he said, 'I found the strength to get out of bed. Your coming has made me feel so much better.' Apparently he had not left his bed for the last four days. The importance he had placed on our visit was quite touching and he insisted on taking us out for a Chinese meal. Arun felt it was unnecessary, and suggested that we order in. Suresh was too ill to go out, but he would have none of that. He got into his wheelchair and we went out for dinner to his favourite Chinese restaurant, fortunately not far from his home.

It is at times like these that the true character of an individual comes through. Suresh knew it was the end of the road for him and yet he was out to spend quality time with us. This encounter was a humbling experience for Arun and gave him a lot of strength, as he talked about it later during his own illness. I do think it helped him deal with his own situation better. They prayed together before we left, knowing fully well that this was the final farewell. The next morning Suresh was to get admitted for blood transfusions.

I was concerned that the dinner had left Suresh too exhausted, so I asked him when we were leaving, 'I hope you didn't overdo it, and will get a good night's sleep.' He smiled and shook his head. There were tears in his eyes as he said, 'I haven't enjoyed a good meal like this in a long while. I wouldn't have sacrificed it for anything.' Content that we had done the right thing in coming to meet him, and that he was not too fatigued, we left their home.

We drove to Penang the next day. 'Penang' means island of the areca nut palms. The countryside was beautiful and green. It was a pleasant drive. We crossed one of the longest bridges in Asia to get to the island. George Town, the old colonial part of Penang, is beautifully maintained, with the new modern city developed around it. This is something I have always admired—progress along with the preservation of the old.

Penang is dominated by the Chinese, and is the most prosperous city in Malaysia. It is famous for its street food. We had some outstanding meals on all four days of our stay, never repeating a dish. Penang Hill, the snake temple, Batu Ferrengi, the orangutans—we saw them all like good tourists. We even managed to go to a typical old colonial club for tea in George Town. This brought back many childhood memories. Satiated with the food and having achieved what we had set out to do, we returned to Delhi.

It had been a hectic trip with air travel, longs walks and long drives. Arun had withstood them all and enjoyed them as well. This shows that a strong mind can uplift the spirits and achieve anything. The strength of mind can take over the body. Suresh had also proved this. What was important for Arun's very being—food, travel, friends and family—had propelled him to forget his own troubles, and live life to the fullest!

Within one month of our return, Suresh passed away. The importance of our visit for Suresh, and its impact on Arun, can never be articulated fully. In many ways, it gave Arun a lot of strength to combat his own disease when the chips were down, to realize that life was too short and whatever needed to be done could not be delayed.

End of the Effectiveness of ADT

Things remained stable till July and Arun continued to work. Honvan, the last of the ADTs, was now failing to keep the PSA down and a fresh bone scan revealed an increase in bony lesions. Arun was progressing to a hormone-resistant form of the disease. From now on he would require chemotherapy. ADT had worked for him for two years and a quarter. We also felt that the homeopathy was not working, so Arun discontinued it. A week later, he read about Tibetan medicine and wanted to try that in addition to chemotherapy. He started taking Tibetan medicine and also learned to meditate.

All through this time, we followed a healthy Indian diet (see p. 19 in 'Grappling with the Diagnosis'). Primarily, it was important to meet Arun's nutritional needs, along with providing any natural preventive supplements that could suppress his cancer in whichever way.

Chemotherapy

The sun is new each day.

—Heraclitus

It was August 2012, and based on the emergence of new bony lesions, it was clear that Arun's disease had progressed despite ADT. Chemotherapy was the new line of treatment proposed. Arun had visited his treating oncologist and they had discussed the risks and benefits of chemotherapy. Out of the range of chemotherapeutic drugs, Docetaxel was selected. It is a first-line drug, used in breast, lung and prostate cancers. It had the best chance of controlling the cancer. Chemotherapy prevents the cancer cells from multiplying by blocking the cancer at particular points in their cell cycle. It manages to contain the disease by preventing cell division.

The date for the start of Arun's chemotherapy was fixed for August 26. This time, we were required to admit him to the hospital for a couple of hours, for the duration of each cycle. So far, we had visited the oncologist in the Out Patient Department (OPD), since most of the treatment had been oral medication, requiring no hospital admission. We opted for day care over a private room for the therapy. The nursing station had a clear view of all its patients and the nurses were prompt to attend to all calls or emergencies. The disadvantage was sharing the space with others. Arun had felt that for a 3–4 hour treatment, this really did not matter.

I had had six cycles of Docetaxel for my cancer, so had prepared Arun according to my experience for his treatment. I gave him a mild purgative and a sleeping pill the night before his chemotherapy. He had an early breakfast of cereal and tea and we left the house by eight. I took an egg and cheese sandwich with some green tea in case he got hungry. I was sure he would not eat the hospital food. It was almost an hour-long drive to the hospital, even that early in the morning.

Day care was rather like an assembly line, with patients on beds or chairs, either lying flat or semi-reclined, side by side, each being fed some toxic medication intravenously. It was Arun's first cycle of chemotherapy, and I was apprehensive about leaving him alone, even for for the admission formalities. But I soon realized, and this was confirmed over time, that for the Malayali nurses he was a VIP (Very Important Person), being from Kerala himself, and I never needed to worry. The nurses identified strongly with him, and addressed him as 'uncle'. Cultural identification helped us in this way.

Arun already had the results of the baseline investigations that were mandatory for the start of each cycle of chemotherapy. As a result, there was no delay in commencing his treatment. All the tests had been in the normal range, barring the rising PSA. The premedication started by ten—it was a cocktail of drugs given to ensure a smooth run of chemotherapy. The Docetaxel drip was started at eleven, and the initial fifteen minutes went slow, to test for any susceptibility or untoward reaction to the medicine. As Arun was comfortable, the speed of medication was then doubled.

Sub-Standard Hospital Food

The usual practice after admission is to address the dietary needs of the patient. I ordered the hospital food just to see what was on offer. Arun was clear he only wanted the sandwich that I had made. The hospital food was unimaginative, all the food items looked similar and not appetizing. Over time I realized that the same fare was doled out at each admission, perhaps for both lunch and dinner. I could see how such mediocre food could be a problem, especially after the many cycles of chemotherapy when one's taste is altered, or in case the patient was required to stay overnight. There was not even a slice of lemon to make the food more palatable.

By 2 pm all was done and we left the hospital for home. The first chemotherapy had gone well. Complications over the next two days were minimal—Arun had a bitter taste in his mouth, minimal nausea, watering from the eyes, constipation and some sleeplessness. Frequent mouth washing helped deal with the first two complications, and a mild purgative over the next two days took care of the constipation. A sleeping pill at night helped him sleep. His appetite returned in a couple of days, and the bone marrow stimulant that was injected ensured normal counts by the end of a week. He had continued to work unhindered during this period.

Interestingly, the bitterness he experienced post-chemotherapy was compounded by the type of food served. He didn't like vegetables and the sight of these always put him off. On the other hand, 'kabab roti' always went down well. I soon realized the need to discuss the daily menu with him before ordering food.

~

> *If music be the food of love, play on, give me excess of it.*
>
> —Shakespeare, *Twelfth Night*

The senses affected most by chemotherapy were taste, smell and, in a way, vision. The constant watering from the eyes interfered with reading over a sustained period of time. As the other senses were intact and heightened to some extent, hearing in particular, I used music to calm his nerves. Aristotle (273–323 BC) wrote about the healing power of music, which we now know helps in pain and chronic depression.[74] Arun enjoyed music and it was effective in distracting him and elevating his mood after chemotherapy.

Even repetitive sounds like the chirping of birds, bubbling of a stream, crackling of a fire and lashing of waves along the shores are all calming. This is nature's soothing symphony. The chirping of birds is common where we live; letting in these sounds in the morning brought the body closer to nature, was pacifying, and promoted tranquillity and serenity. Arun said, 'To wake up to bird sounds gives me an enormous sense of peace, it is the sound of being at home.'

His 'VIP' status in the hospital meant that Arun could slowly make his way to the ward unaccompanied, while I completed the admission formalities before each chemotherapy session. First, I had to collect the admission slip from the oncology OPD on the first floor, then return to the ground floor to pay the treatment advance, and finally proceed to the admissions counter for bed allotment before getting to day care on the fourth floor for the chemotherapy to start. By the time I reached day care, the most proficient phlebotomist, at times coming from the adjacent ward, would have started Arun's drip. He was always allotted bed number 12, the cubicle that was right in front of the nursing station.

Arun's smattering of Malayalam worked like magic, always getting him their full attention. He was one of them and they looked after their own. Us Indians are very parochial but I am not complaining. Arun got special treatment without having to cajole the hospital authorities or a senior doctor. The nurses were very good to the other patients, too. They were sensitive and compassionate, yet we always managed to get the largest cubicle, flooded with natural light, and in full view of the nursing station. Bed number 12 even overlooked a park.

Future Medication Options

Once Arun went on to chemotherapy it was apparent to me that we needed to know all the future options available to us. Surgery, or even standard radiation therapy, both were not feasible options for him. At his stage of the disease, it was important to keep abreast of all the newer developments in cancer research, so that once the newer options became available after FDA approval, we could access them. Treatment in oncology is constantly changing, as knowledge improves—primarily to enhance the effectiveness of the drugs on the cancer cells, but also to reduce the side-effects. To ensure that no stone was left unturned in his treatment, I researched the various new treatment modalities that were being currently developed. At that time, there was a great deal of excitement among medical researchers regarding two new drug trials for prostate cancer.

In the West, prostate cancer is one of the most common malignancies in men over the age of sixty. Hence, researchers are on the constant lookout for a new drug, or a combination of drugs. Most of the research is driven by pharmaceutical companies who are hungry to patent and develop newer medications. The availability of these drugs, even after FDA approval, may be delayed in India for many reasons. One of the newer drugs I found was radioactive, and would have required the Atomic Energy Regulatory Board's approval—not only for the use of the drug but also for the hospital where it could be administered. Such approvals were unlikely to be granted soon enough to benefit Arun, if at all. If we were to consider such a drug for treatment, we would have to travel to the West.

I found that Phase III trials (Phases I and II look at the safety of a drug and its side-effects, while in Phase III clinical trials compare the new drug with the currently available treatments) were being completed for both Abiraterone and Alpharadin at the time. Abiraterone blocks the synthesis of testosterone in all tissues of the body including the tumour (ADT), and could thereby contain the disease by effectively starving the growth and spread of prostate cancer. It was an oral medication and would be available in India soon. Alpharadin (Ra-223), on the other hand, was a type of internal radiotherapy using a radioisotope that worked by delivering minute, highly-charged and targeted doses of damaging radiation to the secondary tumour in the bone.

Radium being similar to calcium (giving strength to the bone), homes in on newly formed bone, thereby delivering radiation to the target. Ra-223 delivers high-energy radiation to small regions, localizing in areas of new bone formation (osteoblastic), as opposed to normal areas of the bone. The bone lesions in prostate cancer are generally osteoblastic. The collateral damage to the normal bone marrow is minimal because the particles have a small range and do not reach the normal bone. This was the drug which required the approval of the Atomic Energy Regulatory Board. Both these newer drugs seemed promising.

We discussed these possibilities with his treating oncologist, who was aware of them but sounded unsure as to how we could arrange for them in India. Alpharadin was his first preference for the next alternative treatment after completing six cycles of chemotherapy.

Arun's disease was mainly in the bones with no visceral involvement (i.e. no other organs were involved), therefore the oncologist's choice was understandable. That evening, after completing the third cycle of chemotherapy, Arun emailed Paul Mathews, who responded promptly and promised that he would get back to him with all the information within the week.

The six cycles of chemotherapy would be completed by the middle of December. So far, things had gone well. Arun had not suffered too much toxicity, but still, a break from chemotherapy was most welcome. Within the Indian scenario, chemotherapy was the only treatment available to him. It gave his body a chance to 'rejuvenate' and regain itself for further therapy in the future.

True to his word, we received a swift response from Paul. His suggestion was to get on to a program on Alpharadin at the Dana Farber Cancer Institute for six cycles, starting in the second week of January. It was appealing and would work perfectly for us. We spoke to Paul and Reji about this proposal and it appeared doable. We worked out the logistics for Arun's stay in Boston at the time of treatment. He could either stay in the US for the entire duration, or return to India after every cycle. Either Adil or I would accompany him during each of the cycles of therapy.

Arun was familiar with Boston—he had spent a year in Cambridge on a Neiman fellowship for journalism at Harvard in 1977. He had subsequently visited the city a number of times while working for *The World Paper*. The idea of spending six months on familiar territory in the US appealed to him. Now, we just had to complete all the formalities. Arun had a valid visa, but I needed to get one. Since we were only in the middle of October, time was on our side.

There was very little red tape in our communications with the Dana Farber Cancer Institute. Most of the formalities were completed online. Arun filled the forms and sent off all the latest investigations—including scans of the x-rays, ultrasound and MRI. The tissue blocks and histopathology slides were sent by courier—they would confirm of Arun's suitability within the next ten days and then we could make the necessary payments. All this was a complete diversion from the treatment Arun was receiving. The fourth cycle of chemotherapy went like a dream—the side-effects were minimal, though he suffered more than the usual fatigue. We dealt with the fatigue by adding a protein drink to increase his protein intake. He managed to eat his three meals adequately with a snack at tea-time.

Just before the fifth cycle of chemotherapy, we got confirmation from the Dana Farber Cancer Institute for

Alpharadin, starting January 16. Reji had offered the use of his home as a base during the treatment. I was hugely relieved that Arun would get a break from chemotherapy and try a drug that was so full of promise. We decided to figure out the logistics of travelling after the first appointment with the doctor and on receiving the first dose of this new drug.

Arun had continued to work and travel during his treatment, making several trips to Lucknow, Bangalore and Bombay. He considered quitting his job before leaving for Boston, but his organization would hear nothing of it and returned his resignation letter. He was told to take a leave of absence, and make a call on resigning only after returning from the US, after the completion of his treatment there. This was fine by him. As long as everything was transparent, there was no question of letting anyone down.

By the middle of December he had completed the last cycle of Docetaxel without much problem. Apparently, the progression of the disease had been halted. Maintaining the dietary requirements during chemotherapy had been a challenge, particularly for the first 4–5 days after the treatment. Steps were taken to overcome these by providing supplements to deal with the possible deficiencies from loss of appetite and inability to eat. Most importantly, it was crucial to maintain a stable weight for a constant dose of chemotherapy.

Travelling to America for Experimental Treatment

Only in the darkness can you see the stars.

—Martin Luther King, Jr.

We left for America, the haven of medical advancement dominated by the pharmaceutical industry, on January 13. We had spent Christmas at home, and even managed a short trip to Bombay to attend a niece's wedding. Delhi had been cold that year, but Boston was freezing. Unsurprisingly, Arun was a bit apprehensive about the trip as he was the worrier in the family. His main concerns were the logistics of our stay during the treatment, rather than the medication itself. I think he felt if he had survived six cycles of chemotherapy, he had the power to overcome any kind of medication—however toxic.

Reji was at the airport to receive us, driving us straight to his home. He had given us his basement flat to stay in. Over the next two days we overcame jetlag and drove around Boston and Cambridge to re-familiarize ourselves with the city we had once lived in. Little had changed as far as the landmarks were concerned, though Hay Market was no longer the bustling place it used to be. The Boston Hospital for Women in Brookline, where I had worked, had disappeared altogether, although the buildings were still there. There were many new restaurants in place of the old ones. But all in all, it was much the same and a manageable city. We met Dr Paul Mathew who had been instrumental in arranging the Ra-223 treatment for Arun.

Ra-223 Treatment

Arun contacted the treatment centre, and was asked to come for a consultation on January 16 at 2 p.m. We were in the hospital by 12.30. After a light lunch in the cafeteria, we slowly made our way to the waiting lounge for the appointment. At 2, we were taken to an unnamed and empty doctor's consultation room. Here we first met a resident doctor who examined Arun and made the case notes. After this, the project in-charge for Alpharadin (Ra-223) took over.

Interestingly, the resident doctor had been a second-generation Indian from Kerala. The senior doctor, on the other hand, was Australian and was interested in the fate of cricket in Australia, especially with respect to the newer forms of the game—T20 and limited overs—where Australia hadn't always fared as well.

He said to Arun: 'There are few side-effects from this treatment. If you develop fever, you need to report back to the hospital. You are required to remain in Boston for five days after receiving the medication, after which you can travel.' When Arun asked about international travel the doctor turned it down, saying, 'Travel is only permitted in America.' He added, 'I haven't been faced with this kind of request earlier, and will discuss it with the rest of the team, and get back to you. Now that you ask, it is logical that if you can travel in America, why not internationally?'Arun considered this a reasonable answer.

We were told to wait for a blood test, and an appointment for the next day's treatment with Ra-223, before leaving. An elderly nurse came to draw the blood sample. She seemed unsure to me; already the skin over a large number of Arun's veins was discoloured from chemotherapy—he didn't have a chemo-port, which is used to administer chemotherapy. We went into the collection room and she poked around, producing two hematomas by counter-puncturing the vein, resulting in collection of blood locally—but failing to draw any blood. She blamed it on thrombosis. I felt she had pre-emptively decided that it was not possible to draw any blood, and so had failed. Usually, venous thrombosis results in cord-like veins which are unlikely to produce hematomas.

Arun was upset with this experience and asked her to stop. I fetched another nurse from the nursing station, explaining the situation to her. She was certainly as proficient as the Malayali nurses he was used to. We were asked to report back to the hospital at 9 the next morning for the medication of Ra-223.

After a quick breakfast of cereal and some excellent coffee at Reji's, we arrived on time for the treatment in the Department of Nuclear Medicine. His blood tests from the previous day were normal. Arun was taken to the treatment room for his injection. The doctor appeared in a biohazard suit for protection against radioactive contamination. The injection was administered rather painlessly, for which Arun was grateful. Fifteen minutes later he was free to go, with a list of precautions.

The precautions were safeguards against pollution by the radioactive waste excreted in the urine and stool. They required proper personal hygiene with multiple rounds of hand-washing and separate washing of used undergarments while wearing gloves to avoid hand contamination. This was necessary for the first forty-eight hours. Drinking lots of fluids to flush out the radioactive waste was also essential.

Now that the first dose of the treatment was over, we needed to take some hard decisions. Fortunately, we got the go-ahead for international travel the next day. It was now clear that Arun could either return to India five days after each dose of Ra-223 or travel within the US. The need to get a flat in Boston was ruled out as Reji generously offered to put Arun up: 'Arun is welcome to stay every month for a week during his treatment.' It was like home for Arun. Both Ann and Reji had been cordial and very hospitable. Ann had cooked many enjoyable meals, and Arun was happy to spend time with their daughter, Amaya. He put up a dramatic performance every morning to get Amaya to drink her milk before school.

We cleared our bill at the hospital, fixed the date for the next treatment, and Arun was told to confirm the date by email before leaving Delhi. The hospital would then order in Ra-223 from Geneva. Each dose was freshly constituted and came specifically for each patient.

Subsequent Rounds of Treatment

I accompanied Arun for the next round of treatment in February, and then again only in April and June. He felt he could manage to remain in America after the second round, travelling to New York and staying with friends. Jetlag had bothered him a bit after returning from the first round. He spent five days with his school friend Amin Aladin, a banker living in New Canaan, reminiscing about school and life in general. Rose, Amin's English wife, had been a teacher—an expert in English Literature—and they had many enjoyable conversations.

Another time, Arun stayed in New York for ten days with Vasanti and Kishore—our friends for thirty-five years—eating home-cooked food and listening to jazz (even going to the Shauman Jazz Bar in Harlem a couple of times). A visit to a priest, Arun's first cousin in Connecticut, after twenty-five years was a high point. Staying on in America had helped Arun reconnect with many friends, and he had been pleased with the opportunity.

Adil had flown in for the March and May treatments—for the third and fifth rounds. He had gone alone for the third round but his wife, Samini, had accompanied him on the second trip. Father and son got on well as people, having similar interests in music and food. Both these rounds had been quite uneventful.

Additional Drugs

When I returned with him in April, the doctors felt the need to add Zytiga to his treatment schedule. To me, this clearly indicated that Ra-223 alone had been effective for only three months. But I was optimistic about the combination. Arun went on to Berkeley to spend time with his cousin, Rohit, and his family, and celebrated his sixty-fifth birthday with them while I returned to Delhi.

While in the Bay area, Arun met with Unni Nair, a college-mate who had undergone a heart transplant and was now restricted to a medical facility. There was certainly no way Unni was ever coming back to India. This visit, though short, did wonders for the morale of both friends. From there, Arun travelled to Maine to meet his father's friends, Judy and Warren Radtke, then on to Florida for the first time to stay with my college friend, Asha, and her husband, Ravi Munshi. Finally, in July he received the last dose of Ra-223, and we returned to Delhi.

For the three months that Arun stayed on in America he received hospitality and immense support from many friends. Each one of them had gone out of their way to welcome him. Arun's illness had truly brought out the best in human nature. Many friends were Indian, but there were others too, including associates he had worked with in America. He had invested well in his friends.

On our journey back after the last round of treatment, Arun asked me whether I thought the Ra-223 had benefitted him—if it had all been worthwhile. I must admit that my expectations had been far greater (the median overall survival was 14 months in the Radium-223 group and 11.2 months in the placebo group). I said, 'The drug was non-toxic. It certainly was effective on its own for three months, and with Zytiga for the next three. So you managed to get off chemotherapy for six months without any pain or increase in the cancer, and travelled in and around America for a bit, meeting friends you otherwise were unlikely to see. Your quality of life was great. I think it was certainly worth it.'

Arun agreed with my observations.

Developing Drug Resistance

I love those who can smile in trouble.

—Leonardo da Vinci

Restarting Chemotherapy

In August 2013, we returned to my husband's oncologist, Dr AA. He wanted Arun to restart chemotherapy while continuing with Zytiga. He also felt Zytiga alone would not contain the disease. He prescribed Docetaxel for the next three months, in three weekly cycles as before. The doctors found evidence of disease progression in October, and a change in chemotherapy was warranted. Fortunately for Arun, the medication was oral this time round. He only had to get blood tests every three weeks and a bone scan at the end of three months, the reports of which were to be sent to the oncologist. So far, all oral medication had always worked well. It was painless to administer and easy to transport while travelling.

Arun continued to work, walk, and travel as before. His appetite remained good, maintaining a healthy Indian diet. We managed to do a family trip to Coonoor for Christmas that year. Flying to Coimbatore and driving up to Coonoor the next morning, it was as close to nature as you could get. There were rolling tea gardens on either side of the road and the Nilgiris were lush and green—soothing to the tired eyes of the plain-dwellers of north India. Arun was content to have uninterrupted quality time with his grandchildren.

Later, we went on a road trip to Bharatpur in February 2014 so that the grandchildren could see the large migratory birds that come to India every year. The three-day trip proved very fruitful for the adults, although the children found it difficult to focus on the birds—either nesting or hiding in the bushes—from long distances. The children were fascinated by the snakes at the bird sanctuary and the peacocks that woke us up every morning at our hotel, The Bagh. They were regulars at the Delhi Zoo, going there almost once every three months, and remained fascinated by the large caged animals, but observing birds from long distances was a different story.

Rising PSA and Repeated Drug Resistance

After we returned, we discovered that Arun's PSA was rising. It was becoming apparent that while some chemotherapy had worked for three–four months, the rest only manifested in toxicity and no benefit. Why was drug resistance occurring repeatedly with so many of the treatments that Arun had received? To begin with, he developed resistance to Casodex and the other hormone-blocking drugs. This was followed by resistance to Ra-223, and then to Zytiga and Docetaxel. Drug resistance was proving to be the cause of therapeutic failure at regular intervals and relapse of the disease. Was the cancer outsmarting his body's ability to curtail it while still on a particular anti-cancer drug (See p. 38–40 in 'Drug Resistance')?

In view of Arun's rising PSA, his oncologist suggested we start Xtandi, a new drug, which was recently approved by the FDA and had become available internationally—although it had yet not arrived in India. In March 2014, it was prescribed to Arun and we had to get special permission from the Ministry of Health to import this medicine. Though the drug was orally administered, Arun had a great deal of toxicity with this therapy, including nausea and fatigue. Besides, it did little to control his disease and the oncologist decided to stop this treatment within two months. It was ineffective. The PSA had continued to rise during the two months of the new medication.

The Sense of Touch

Tumors are wounds that do not heal. Every cancer medication should improve wound healing.

—Rudolph Virchow

With the failure of Xtandi, Arun's fatigue continued to increase slowly but steadily. It was becoming too difficult for him to continue working, and he wanted to spend the time he had left in pursuit of things that gave him the most pleasure. In May 2014, he resigned from his job. He also stopped taking Tibetan medicine and switched to Ayurvedic treatment.

Ayurvedic Treatment

The Kottakkal group for Ayurvedic medicine has a hospital in East Delhi. There we met a young, articulate doctor, who gave us a prescription for three medicines. One was to boost the immune system, the second was a 'churnam' for detoxification and the third was a medicated oil for massaging the areas of pain. He clearly stated that there was no drug in their arsenal that could target the cancer cells directly; he also reassured us that none of the medicines he had prescribed contained heavy metals or would interfere with the chemotherapy.

We started the Ayurvedic medicines in May. All the prescribed medicines seemed completely logical—the immune system boost would help fight the cancer from within, while detoxification was necessary to remove the destroyed cancer cells and any other waste material that had accumulated in the body after chemotherapy. Earlier, we had given Arun purgatives whenever the need arose, but now they were administered daily. The immediate fallout of this was an improvement in appetite and some reduction in his fatigue.

Importance of Touch

Every evening, before bedtime, I gave Arun a light massage with the prescribed Ayurvedic oil on the lower back and left hip—these were the areas where the pain had first begun. The massages had more than one effect. Firstly, the medicine in the oil was therapeutic; secondly, the act of touching had a calming effect on Arun. Maybe, massages reassure the patient that the caregiver is committed to their well-being. The gentle rubbing signals your concern and makes the patient more serene. This may be the true essence of Ayurvedic massages—telling the patient they are still alive and that you are there for them. The massage is a tactile way of expressing love.

We receive tactile information from the world around us every day and it is central to our lives. We have two touch systems—the discriminating and the emotional touch system. Early touch experiences are important for the development of both cognitive functions and a healthy body.[75] The skin, a membrane that covers the entire body, is perhaps our largest organ through which we communicate with the world outside.

The experience of the movements we make, the textures and the people we touch, are the first joys of life itself. The immediate tranquillity of a mothers' touch—being held and fed by her—is ingrained in our minds from birth. This tactile experience is the earliest form of communication, from the time we gain consciousness. In other words, we live by the sense of touch. Adam Gopnik's observation about touch: 'What we see we long for; what we hear we interpret; what we touch we are,' may well be true after all.[76]

This remarkable insight is even more pronounced in team sport. When players touch one another and acknowledge a good shot or performance, their morale is much higher than those players who are aloof and individualistic. Touch lowers stress, builds morale, and produces oneness that helps teams to triumph. The same applies to sick patients. **A gentle massage in the area of pain, with or without oil, can be soothing.**

Continued Drug Resistance

In May Arun was started on a new drug, Carboplatin, and in July, Navelbine was added to his medication. Arun was steadily getting resistant to more and more drugs. Our concerns continued to mount as the options available to us slowly dwindled. We had already exhausted the newer drugs for prostate cancer which had only recently been approved by the FDA and introduced into the market. Besides, Arun was alone at home while I continued to work. I realized that I needed to rid myself of the stresses of work and dedicate more time to his well-being. The time we had left together was getting shorter as the days went by, so I resigned from my job.

Discussions about Life and Death

Love begins at home, and it is not how much we do... but how much love we put in the action.

—Mother Teresa

Arun wanted me to continue working because I enjoyed it so much, but in August 2014, I quit. His physical decline was apparent—I needed to spend more time with him. There was no point in repenting later. I had always believed that whatever was worth doing, had to be in service of the living.

We had been married for forty-one years. I had met Arun while doing my internship in Delhi in 1972. Most doctors usually marry doctors and feel okay about creating a hospital scenario even at home—'A hospital away from the hospital,' is how I liked to describe it. But I thought that that was going too far. It had always been clear to me that I could never marry a doctor. The doctor couples whom I knew had doctor friends, and thus, their social lives centred around medicine and doctoring. There must have been a great sense of security in that, but, to me, it seemed that there was no other dimension to their lives.

Profession and family for me were two separate arenas with no meeting ground. The home scene *had* to be different. I was already a doctor and worked with similar people—the idea of a doctor for a spouse was too dull. My life had to be different. I had done little but study after leaving school—first for my undergraduation and then for my postgraduate degree. Arun and I were the same age. After a postgraduate degree in English, he had taken time off to hitchhike through Europe for a year, before joining his first job as a reporter at *The Indian Express*. I, on the other hand, still needed to complete a specialization before I could think of doing anything meaningful. The days of success with a simple MBBS degree were long over.

Ours was a marriage with a lot of understanding, best described as happy. We had our different professional pursuits which never entered the home—a tranquil place for the family. We gave each other space to do the things that mattered the most to each of us. Arun liked travelling and socializing while I liked to read. Both of us also enjoyed spending time with the family. Family holidays were times of complete togetherness.

Arun was many things—his surname was typically Syrian Christian, but he was born in Kanpur, and schooled in Kanpur as well as in Nainital. His college education was in Delhi and Lucknow. He looked like a 'cut Sardar' to the north Indian, a Pathan in Pakistan, 'one of them' in Kerala, spoke Lukhnawi Urdu, and his most favourite food was Mughlai. He enjoyed Sufi music along with jazz. Despite his name, he could easily claim antecedents from anywhere in India. At the time I met him, he was the antithesis of my father—a retired army general who was rather prim and proper. When we first met he was in the kurta-pajama phase of his life. He wore chappals, kept a beard and had long hair that curled behind his ears. He was completely different from anyone I had met before.

Our disagreements were few. His major 'flaw' was his punctuality, even though it did not matter in our context. In Delhi, everyone was late. Some friends even arrived at a party after dinner was served. But Arun was never late for an invite, often arriving before the host or hostess appeared. His insistence on punctuality was annoying at the time, especially when he showed irritation at a five-minute delay on my part. Before I could start getting ready to go out, he would enter my room, banging at my door and then pacing noisily outside till I emerged. We were still the first to arrive in any case. The whole show was predictable, even amusing sometimes. I realized early on in my married life that this was unnecessary friction—Arun never wanted to lose social time with his friends—and I learned not to take those extra five minutes, even after a long day at work.

All in all, it was a marriage that worked. Our son was the proof—always relaxed and happy to be home. We got on well, both collectively and individually, and travelled together extensively. We discussed all the important issues and found solutions through open discussions. Nobody was ever out of the loop. We were from three different professions—a journalist, a doctor and a wealth manager—but as a family we were one.

By the end of September, Arun started on Cabazitaxel and Carbozantinib after the previous combination had failed. While the former, a semi-synthetic taxoid, was similar to Docetaxel, Carbozantinib inhibited the enzyme tyrosine kinase, which reduced tumour growth, metastasis and blood vessel formation. This was the last combination of conventional drugs for prostate cancer. He tolerated this treatment well.

A Necessary Conversation

We managed to spend quality time together, discussing outstanding issues, including questions about life and death. We all need to have these conversations with our loved ones. It helps everyone deal better with the situation. We had made all of our lives' decisions jointly and freely—there was no reason for the discussions about death to be taboo. At the best of times this can be difficult and emotional. Very often, these conversations left me with an overwhelming sense of loneliness.

Death is not a dirty word. We need to talk about it. Anything born or living will eventually die. It is inevitable. And yet, this topic is never discussed. We prepare for the birth of a child in every which way. For instance, the mother is taught breathing exercises to help with pain during labour, helping her prepare for the pain to come. The husband is often a part of these preparations—she is not alone. Similarly, prior to surgery, every detail is discussed by the surgeon, just like in chemotherapy. The patient is made aware of all the likely complications and how to counter them. So then, why do we not talk about and prepare for death? Being open with each other about death could ease the anxiety and the fear surrounding it.

For us, the question was: how could Arun's life be prolonged without compounding his suffering. The apprehension about what would happen was immense. When one is terminally ill, with little or no prospects beyond the agony and disability of the disease, should one not have the right to die? There is no way around the argument for dying with dignity.

Euthanasia

It is the patient's autonomy to make such personal choices, considering the hopelessness (or hopefulness) of the situation they find themselves in. The right to refuse medical treatment is well recognized in law, and this includes treatment that sustains life—i.e. passive euthanasia. Within this law, the removal of life-supporting treatment in the face of imminent death, as well as do-not-resuscitate are both included.

Active euthanasia is illegal in India and remains a distant dream. But it has been prevalent in many countries in Europe, with the earliest adoption by the Netherlands.[77] Oregon became the first state in the US to legalize physician-aided suicide in 1997 with the Death with Dignity Act.[78] This law requires the approval of two doctors and confirmation by two witnesses. The doctors must agree that the patient is of sound mind and doesn't have more than six months to live.

No one wants to see needless suffering. Caring for the dying, even in the medical profession, is a profoundly difficult task. It is devastating for the caregiver, who faces the biggest challenge—providing a satisfactory quality of life. When all efforts to eliminate the physical, psychological and social stress have failed, what then? Why should suffering be 'carried forward' when there is no cure? It is true that patients with social support and close family connections fare better with the stresses of their illness.[79] The desire to hasten death only surfaces when there is loss of dignity, poor quality of life and the perception of being a burden on others. The solution lies in understanding the underlying problem and addressing it in an appropriate manner.

In India, this conundrum has been partially addressed. On March 9, 2018 in a landmark ruling, the Supreme Court of India made it legal for a 'terminally-ill individual to decline use of life support measures, allowing families of those in incurable coma to withdraw such measures to reduce the period of suffering, thereby permitting patient's euthanasia.'[80] The court also recognized the right of a living will—clearly spelling out one's wishes regarding medical treatment—made by a terminally-ill individual. A 'living will', made by a patient of sound mind, takes away the painful burden of such a decision from a family member. This right to live and die with dignity gives the patient a chance to spend their final hours or days with their loved ones—not in a hospital bed but at home.

Arun often asked me how he was doing and how much time he had left. I had no answer—I had often kept quiet. It was not that I was unaware of his anxiety or his predicament, but I didn't know how to address it. Finally, after much thought I explained the situation to him: 'Yes, you are short on treatment options as most of the drugs tried so far are ineffective because of drug resistance, but while these current medicines work, there is still hope. You have no pain and can still do all the things important to you—you need to relish the time left, we all do!' It was not as if Arun was unaware of all this, but he needed the assurance that all was well at that time.

Moving on to Palliative Care

How can you hide from what never goes away?

—Heraclitus

Through January and February 2015, Arun had his last two cycles of chemotherapy. In the beginning of January the pain had returned. The reappearance of pain was a sign of disease progression. He now needed round-the-clock pain medication to keep him comfortable. It was evident that, in spite of the chemotherapy being given, his disease was getting the upper hand. Further treatment would be ineffective and unlikely to benefit him.

Arun's worst fear had returned. The pain brought with it intense suffering. Around the time of the last chemotherapy session in February, he had breakthrough pain with no relief from the pain medication. As a result, a pain patch was added to the oral pain medicine he was taking round-the-clock. The endeavour now was to provide complete pain relief. With the addition of the pain patch, his discomfort disappeared and he was at ease.

Non-conventional Treatment

He had come to the end of the line with the known conventional chemotherapeutic drugs, so we tried non-conventional treatment. He was given a new drug, Avastin, which blocked new blood vessel formation—essential for the nutritional needs of a spreading cancer—in an attempt to see if it would somehow halt the progress of the disease. These drugs were usually prescribed for the treatment of other malignant tumours—not prostate cancer.

However, this trial proved futile and the PSA continued to rise during both these cycles of chemotherapy. The bone scan also registered an increase in the number of lesions. As the tumour relentlessly continued to replace the bone marrow, he required blood and platelet transfusion. Clearly, it was growing unchecked.

These new drugs were given on the assumption that they would suppress all rapidly proliferating cells by interfering with the blood supply of the growing tumour. The primary target was the tumour in the bone, though secondarily, the normal cells of the bone marrow were also taking a hit—an unavoidable collateral damage. It turned out to be a double-blow—the tumour was replacing the bone marrow while the chemotherapy was suppressing production of the normal blood cells. Therefore, blood and platelet transfusions became a necessity, along with stopping the chemotherapy. This was the only way forward now. The body had endured a lot, trying to cope with the ravages of the disease in the form of bone metastasis. Added to this was the burden of marrow destruction—the side-effect of the treatment.

These last two cycles of non-conventional chemotherapy had been difficult. The described toxicity for these chemotherapeutic drugs was upsetting—there was bleeding from the nose and mouth due to low platelet counts. This added further stress on the bone marrow, which was already stretched thin. Blood loss triggers bone marrow proliferation, but where was the marrow? It was being destroyed by the tumour and being suppressed by the treatment. Fortunately, these episodes of bleeding lasted only for three days. As the effect of the transfusion kicked in, the bleeding stopped. With medications prescribed in the discharge summary and multiple small meals, Arun was kept hydrated and nourished.

Arun said to me, 'I did the last two rounds because I did not want to disappoint any one, not my friends or family and particularly not you, Arati. It has been hard for me, but I did it all the same. I don't think this is really working and this is not really living. I can't enjoy anything anymore—not the food I eat, not even my grandchildren, as I am constantly feeling unwell. I have had a good life so far and have no regrets. Death is inevitable now. Let's leave it up to God... The stage has come to call it quits. Look at what it is doing to my body! It is not worth the struggle. It is a losing battle.'

End of Chemotherapy

Arun had been squeamish about blood and wary of needles all his life, but the two and a half years of chemotherapy had changed him as a person. All these adversities that he had overcome had made him very brave. This inner strength must have come from his desire to not let anyone down. But it was now obvious to him that he was unlikely to gain from any further chemotherapy. Besides, it was adding to his misery and creating unnecessary complications. Arun wanted to stop all treatment and go on to supportive care.

We talked to his treating oncologist, who agreed that the treatment had failed. He admitted, 'All three parameters that have been used to monitor him throughout his therapy are clearly showing progression of disease and failure of chemotherapy.' We consulted other oncologists in Delhi, as well as our friend in Boston, Dr Paul Mathews, who had participated in so many of our decisions. Everyone was on the same page. The time had come to stop chemotherapy and move on to palliative care.

Shifting to Palliative Care

Two weeks after stopping the treatment, Arun felt better. He managed to eat more per meal, so we reduced the number of meals from eight to six per day. He could do short walks from the house to the gate—about fifty meters—twice a day. He was back to visiting the grandchildren every afternoon. However, he could no longer navigate the stairs and used the lift instead to get to their second-floor apartment.

A palliative care team from CanSupport visited Arun.

It comprised of a doctor, a nurse, and a social worker. There was no priest. They visited once a month, but were a phone call away when the need arose, welcoming telephonic discussion at any time. This was an ideal arrangement, reassuring to the patient and to the caregiver without being intrusive. All three visitors were cheerful, with a ready smile, and were always willing to lend an ear. They assessed many things in the home and the diet, and gave tips to improve the quality of care being given to the patient. Arun was always reassured by this interaction. For the pain, he consulted a specialist in pain management. Mostly, the medication kept the pain in check.

As his illness progressed he sought comfort from the Church. He made contact with two priests. This resulted in a home visit by one of them. Once they realized that his condition was steadily declining and he was unable to come to church, the priests kept in telephonic contact and made one or two visits per month.

Reverend Winston Samuel—one of the priests who visited—was himself suffering from cancer, and was on palliative care. His own affliction did not deter him from making these visits and providing comfort to another. His visits gave Arun a great deal of strength and solace. The other priest, Dr Paul Swarup, was quite articulate, often talking at length with Arun. Comforting patients through sickness at home should be a social obligation for all priests, and without financial implications.

Careful planning, with an understanding of the processes involved, ensured that Arun's weight loss was limited to 5 kilos during the five years of treatment—mostly occurring during chemotherapy. Arun did not develop cachexia (the wasting syndrome associated with cancer or other chronic diseases). He had eaten two eggs daily, apart from meat, fish or poultry, which was consumed once a day during palliative care. Additional protein supplements were added to the milk or juice, whose vitamins had also benefited him. His taste had improved greatly and he no longer had anorexia or nausea.

Arun realized that he had come to the end of the road. He had short spurts of energy which he utilized to enjoy meeting friends and family and eating out. However, travelling, which had been an integral part of his life, crucial to his quality of life, was now out of the question. At the end of March, we celebrated our son, Adil's, birthday. This was possibly the last meal which Arun ate outside.

His daily visits to the grandchildren were also becoming difficult. By the first week of April, he could manage two visits a week and these, too, left him very tired. One night, even though there were grab rails, he was unable to get off the commode unaided. It took a great deal of effort on my part to help him back to bed. My major concern had always been that a fall in his condition could result in a fracture of his diseased hip. It was inevitable that help would be required at night, so the next day I arranged for a night attendant to help him with the stiffness in his legs.

On May 1, we celebrated his sixty-seventh birthday at home, with my brother and his family. Arun wanted to eat Chinese food. He attended his party in a wheelchair, sat and interacted with everyone for about an hour, ate some dinner, cut the cake and returned to his room, quite exhausted.

By now, he was also developing an enormous amount of anxiety. Some of it was related to his expected demise, but that he could mostly take in his stride. Rather, most of his apprehensions were related to the family members, those that he was leaving behind. Arun had been a journalist, sensitive to the changing scenario in India and the general state of unrest in the country. The level of social unrest around the country in 2014-15 was something we had not really witnessed in our growing-up years. The complete intolerance and polarization that was taking place in society made the minorities unsure and insecure—he had Muslim friends and was a Christian himself. All this was apparently invisible to the ruling elites but it bothered him to no end. He often wondered, with the rising communal turmoil, what the future held for our grandchildren.

Haematuria and the Growing Tumour

Towards the end of May he developed haematuria (blood in the urine) at six a.m. one morning. I realized that he required hospitalization. The oncology centre, which he had previously attended for his chemotherapy, was at least an hour's drive from home, provided the Delhi traffic was light. Arun was practical and felt that since admission was a distinct possibility, we should try and find a hospital in the vicinity of our home. A surgeon colleague of mine suggested a multi-speciality hospital ten minutes away and promised to speak to the urologist there.

We arrived in casualty and were immediately attended to by a young consultant in urology. He was efficient, and started a bladder wash in no time, removing the clots and establishing the free flow of urine. Arun was admitted and formalities completed by ten. Things were beginning to settle down. Blood needed to be arranged—the donors had arrived and I went to the blood bank to request for fresh blood so that Arun could get the maximum benefit from the transfusion.

Blood is normally separated into its components in the blood bank. These components, depending on the patient's requirements, are then transfused. In this way, the same unit of blood can benefit more than one patient. Arun's requirement was for red blood cells and platelets. As platelets have a short shelf life, these are invariably given fresh. The red blood cells, on the other hand, have a longer shelf life of up to forty-two days. Understandably, as the blood ages, the senescent red cells are destroyed. Therefore, the transfusion of older blood is likely to be less effective. In Arun's condition, the fresher the blood the longer it was likely to sustain his needs. He had developed anaemia for two reasons: marrow replacement by tumour and the blood loss because of haematuria.

It was obvious that, by now, the tumour was growing unchecked and had infiltrated the urinary bladder—causing obstruction leading to the retention of urine, infection and haematuria. In palliative care, the treatment is supportive, taking care of symptoms as they develop. In Arun's case it involved removing the obstruction, controlling the infection and replacing the blood loss.

So far Arun had taken every day as it had come, but during this admission he became completely disoriented. The stay in the hospital weakened him greatly. Far from restoring his health, he got sicker and lost the will to fight his disease. He remained in the hospital for three nights. Though his problem settled, and the urine cleared, we found him unwilling to stay on.

Arun was not one to complain, but something had changed during this admission. It seemed like the spark had gone out of his eyes. His desire to continue the fight against cancer was no longer there. He felt claustrophobic and incarcerated in the hospital. As soon as his condition was stable enough for me to manage him myself, I brought him home on a catheter and on antibiotics.

The Last Mile

Neither the sun nor death can be looked at steadily.

—La Rochefoucauld

And now the end is near,
And so I face the final curtain.
My friends, I say it clear
I state my case of which I am certain.
I have lived a life that's full,
I travelled each and every highway,
And more, much more than that, I did it my way.

—'My Way', Frank Sinatra

Arun had—for forever and a day—done things his way. This was the story of his life, therefore Sinatra's song is appropriate here. In any case, he had always enjoyed listening to it when the chips were down.

He had wanderlust. Much to his parents' horror, their only son had taken off to travel across Europe with one hundred dollars in his pocket, right after his Master's. He had some traveller's cheques in his father's name but he was unsure whether these were encashable. This did not deter him from making the trip. He had a burning desire to travel. Twenty-four countries later, and after thirteen months on the move, he described his experience as 'Meaningful…more educative than any formal education I could have got. It prepared me well for later life.'

Coming home from hospital was a huge relief to him. He wanted to eat chicken biryani, raita and salad for his first dinner after discharge. I had arranged oxygen in case the claustrophobia he had felt in the hospital returned. Earlier, he had help in the form of a night attendant, now he had assistance in the day-time as well. He was largely confined to the wheelchair. His blood pressure fell periodically while attempting to stand.

He went back to as much of his daily routine as he could. He was again having eight small meals, meeting friends between five and six every evening, and sitting in his favourite place in the house—the interior garden—watching the birds. The garden was frequented by the sun bird and the Indian robin. He had named a pair of Indian robins after his grandchildren, Arman and Seher. Every day, after having spotted them, he was content to move back to his room and into air-conditioned comfort.

Both the grandchildren were now in regular school. Their mother made an effort to bring the children to visit with him at least twice a week. By now, Arun had weakened considerably, and could only manage about fifteen minutes of quality time and appreciating their playfulness.

Both the priests came on different occasions to meet with him over the next ten days. Arun had clarified his position with both of them regarding the funeral. It was June and exceedingly hot. As it would take the better part of twenty four-hours for us to get the permission for the burial, he had decided on a cremation first, followed by burial of the ashes. He wanted both of these last rites to be presided over by the priests. It was reassuring when both of them agreed to this, informing us that this was not an unusual request, but rather a rising trend.

Ever since his discharge from the hospital at the end of May, Arun had been under constant supervision in a manageable, though slowly declining state. The cancer had started with pain, but the pain associated with dying had an unimaginable intensity. Arun's disease had predominantly been in the bone. 'My bones feel like they are exploding,' was how he described it. It was tumour-related pain but it was aggravated by anxiety.

Keeping him pain-free during this period had become a major challenge. Too much pain medicine left him drowsy and sleepy all day, too little brought on the pain. It was difficult to strike the perfect balance. He was on round-the-clock pain medicine and a pain patch, whose dose had steadily increased over the last few weeks. Also, there was oral morphine for whenever there was breakthrough pain.

On June 13 he wanted to eat appam and stew for lunch. He ate this with great relish—the satisfaction visible on his face. At two in the morning the emergency bell rang in my room. As I entered Arun's room, the night attendant met me near the door. He said, apologizing, 'Sahib wants to talk to you urgently. He is restless and not able to sleep.' I approached Arun's bed, turned on the oxygen and then sat beside him, holding his hand.

He was silent for a while and then he said, 'Arati, you are holding me back. You need to let me go. I can't live like this anymore—my life is meaningless. I don't want resuscitation. Don't take me to any hospital, not again.'

I reassured him and said, 'I will keep you at home. You need to relax, breathe deeply, and be at peace with yourself. Try and get some sleep.' I sat with him for an hour. We did breathing exercises together for five minutes—this relaxed him, and ten minutes later he was asleep.

Advancement in medical science has made great strides in the treatment and cure for various diseases. It has greatly increased longevity. As a result, sometimes the duration of life outweighs the quality of life. It was quality of life that Arun had always hankered for—meeting friends, eating good food and travelling. These were slowly being denied him because of his slowly but steadily deteriorating health from the spreading cancer. For him, this was not prolonging life, but prolonging agony.

He was apparently now prepared for the final eventuality. Was this his way of telling me that the end was near? We all need to have conversations about death with our loved ones. Death is inevitable. He wanted to die at home and not hooked up to a ventilator, or with food being pumped into his veins. For him, this was the happier alternative, and our duty as a family was to give all the love and necessary comfort to him at home. Adil had moved back to the house to spend as much time as possible with his father in his final hours.

Two days later, Adil gave him his protein-rich drink at noon. Arun said he needed to nap. An hour later, his respiration became laboured and at two in the afternoon he had left us.

~

Grief was the celebration of love, those who could feel real grief were lucky to have loved.

—Chimamanda Ngozi Adichie

We are all human and life is precious to all of us. A sudden unexpected death comes as a shock. However, even an expected death is painful. The void created in either type of death is similar, and palpable. Though the suffering was finally over for him, the emptiness he had left behind was profound.

Six months later, Arman and Seher still come every day at about five in the evening to the internal garden.

Friendships and Remembrances

Piglet sidled up to Pooh from behind.
'Pooh!' he whispered.
'Yes, Piglet?'
'Nothing,' said Piglet, taking Pooh's paw.
'I just wanted to be sure of you.'

—A.A. Milne, *The House at Pooh Corner*

A friend is someone who knows about you and still loves you.

—Elbert Hubbard

This narrative would be incomplete if I did not talk about Arun's friends. Arun was a people's person. I often felt that his brain was wired differently, recording every detail of a previous meeting, however long ago it may have been. He could recall each event, as if it had happened just yesterday. I often wondered whether this had something to do with his Malayali genes.

Kerala is an emerald in the Indian crown—its radiant countryside is beautiful. I have always found it unnerving to see how Arun, who was originally from Kurainnoor, and his family were so connected to each other—including all extended family and distant cousins. It is strangely fascinating too, how on just a mention of your family name, it would not be unusual for your antecedence to be laid out before you, reconnecting you to your past. You are freshly re-hooked to your family tree in the matter of an evening, without any difficulty. The Syrian Christians have made genealogy into an art form. Even though many of them have migrated to other places, they haven't lost this skill. Arun had never lived in Kerala, but he had achieved the same expertise in this art form, successfully applying it to all the people he knew in north India.

The Isolation of Cancer

Cancer is a serious illness and a long journey that is completely isolating. What sustains you in this journey is the love and concern of family and friends, who help alleviate the loneliness, diminish anxiety and other symptoms related to emotional distress. They provide the anchor to weather any storm.

Many things happen when you have cancer, some of which are unexplainable. Only a few people empathize with your situation, but most offer no feelings at all and some even begin to avoid you. Still others, who were once considered close not so long ago, drop you completely. The question that arises then is: what happened? Are human relationships so fickle? Why did they change? Did the person become discernibly different because he had cancer? These were troubling questions in troubled times.

I recall an incident when Arun was to meet a friend for lunch in Goa. Another visitor to Goa, a common 'friend' also visiting from Delhi, rang Arun's host and immediately got invited to join in. After finding out about Arun, he refused to come, saying, 'Are you aware how sick he is? Meeting someone that sick kills joy.' This person was an ex-colleague whom Arun had known his entire working life. They had both joined *The Indian Express* as reporters around the same time.

I have wondered a lot about this phenomenon wherein people start avoiding sick people. Perhaps they become aware of their own vulnerability, avoiding such a stark reminder. Perhaps it is a fear that cancer may somehow be transmitted. It could even be a part of the moral degradation that has happened in India, where human relationships have taken such a tumble. Or is it that with your deadly disease, you have already lost the right to live, and therefore the right to exist as a friend?

Knowing how much Arun valued his friends, I wondered

if they wanted to talk about him with me. I was pleased when some of them expressed interest in sharing their stories and memories of Arun. For me, it was a good way to learn about aspects of Arun's personality that I as a spouse was unaware of.

There are many facets to each individual. How a person appears to an outsider depends entirely on which facet she experiences. The face seen by a friend may be quite different from the one viewed by a spouse. We were good friends, Arun and I, and got on well together as people, but I was also his wife. As I see it, there is openness in friendship with no inhibitions or liabilities. Friendship, in a way, is pure. You seldom have to justify yourself, there are no preconceptions, and there is an intimate understanding, sometimes without having to utter a word. These facets a spouse is never privy to. The bonds with friends are based on memories and not on genetics or marriage. A friends' perception comes without bias and is therefore unique. How did his friends view him?

Arun had a strong sense of loyalty towards his friends, sometimes without reason. When some friend did not visit him as his health declined, all he ever said was, 'I am disappointed. He was a close friend.'

He kept in touch with most of the people he had known throughout his life and travels, often across continents. Surprising though it may seem, he even had close bonds with people from his kindergarten days. Even when a friend moved to another city, Arun had remained in touch. These were the days of no cell phones, rarely available landlines, and no computers or emails—only 'snail mail'. Keeping in touch was a mammoth task, but Arun had kept up with the parents of his friends. In fact, this is how I had met him. He was my older brother's friend from college and used to visit my parents often. In the following pages, I have combined the different accounts of Arun from his friends, so that he may be visualized as a complete person.

Arun Through his Friends' Eyes

Sandy Shaw

Arun was an only child. The closest thing he had to a sister was Sandy Shaw. Sandy had migrated to Australia soon after finishing school in the mid-sixties, returning to India only a few years ago. Arun had kept in touch with her for all those years and visited with her in Goa at least twice a year. It was Sandy who had compelled him to use the wheelchair on his return journey from Goa in January 2015—his last trip out of Delhi. He had struggled getting in at the Delhi airport, but had refused any help.

'It makes me feel like an invalid,' he had said.

Sandy visited him in April 2015, before things really deteriorated. This is what she had to say later, after Arun was gone:

> I don't know where to start to write about my dear friend Arun, someone I have known for over five decades and, more importantly, someone who has been a cherished part of my life.
>
> There are only a handful of people that pass through this pathway of life that you can call a real friend—someone who cares for you, who is genuinely interested in how your life is panning out without being overly curious, who is always in the wings, in case you have a real fall. Arun was that friend to me.
>
> He was a gentle person at heart. He always tried to catch up with his numerous friends while he was travelling. Somehow we remained in touch over all these years, touching base with a Christmas card or a phone call from around the world. Distance never interfered between us.
>
> Arun was a bit apprehensive about my return to India in my retirement years. He was only satisfied that I had done the right thing after a visit to Goa. He was happy with my surroundings and friends, and felt that I would be safe.
>
> I am so glad I visited Arun when I did, as I felt he had

endured enough suffering. I needed to say goodbye to him. Appropriately, on my last visit, he wanted the Anglican priest to visit his home, and we took holy communion together. It was then that I knew I wouldn't see him again.

Rohit Salve

Arun loved children, and Rohit Salve—a cousin who was younger to him by ten years—was the first baby he had ever held. He had always loved Rohit dearly for having permitted him that ecstatic moment, and not howling in his arms. Rohit wrote:

> My first recollection of Arun is from the mid-1970s, when he appeared at our home in Kalimpong—bearded, long-haired, clad in pajama-kurtha and with a rucksack draped over his back. Barely a teenager then, I remember opening the door to this stranger, my cousin, who looked like a hippie/Jesus Christ. How cool was that?
>
> Since then, as a series of tragic events unfolded in our family, I became increasingly aware of Arun as a member of my family. However, it was only after my father suddenly died, that Arun became an immediate presence in my life, providing the radar to a boat that could have easily run aground in the smallest of storms.
>
> As I look back to those years of a young college student in India, and some of the particularly poor choices I made, I recall him stepping in and bailing me out, while remaining completely non-judgmental. It is ironic, that while we initially crossed paths because of misfortune, we had thirty-five rich years together as Arun transitioned from being a father-figure to a friend.
>
> When I think about Arun, I see the solid blocks that made the core of his foundation—compassion, integrity, curiosity...and I see his unwavering faith in God. I am grateful that he stepped into my life, and that we wove a beautiful tapestry together. I am thankful that my children and wife were, through Arun, able to get glimpses of a wonderful grandfather and father-in-law they never met.

And I am very proud that the cool and classy Arun was my friend.

The largest contingent of Arun's friends were from Pakistan. As a journalist he had covered Pakistan extensively in the eighties and nineties. He said about Pakistan: 'It is the one country I always felt most welcome. I was as much at home there as I am in India. My experiences in Pakistan were always memorable. Besides, I enjoyed their food.'

Zohra Yusuf

One of his closest friends was Zohra Yusuf, a former editor of *The Star Weekend*, now a freelance journalist and advertising executive. She is also Chairperson of the Human Rights Commission of Pakistan. She became a family friend over the years, and has remained in touch even after he passed away. Zohra wrote:

> I had heard of Arun shortly before meeting him. I think it was sometime in autumn 1983, when I received several telexes from the editor of *World Paper*, Boston, expressing concern for his safety as an Indian journalist who was scheduled to visit Pakistan. I was working as the editor of *The Star Weekend* which carried the *World Paper*—Arun was one of its international editors. While I mulled over what we could possibly do, considering we had no contact details, Arun had arrived in Karachi over the weekend, visited the press club and had already made friends and useful professional contacts—even before we had met.
>
> I think it was his winning smile when he walked into my office that quickly made us friends. But there were many other friends that he soon made in Pakistan. An outgoing, easy-going person with a natural journalistic curiosity, Arun had the knack of putting people at ease even as he extracted all the information he needed—either for a story or for a deeper understanding of Pakistan and the issues that concerned him. Though gentle in his ways, he had a

hard nose for stories and pursued them relentlessly. His persistence usually paid off. Through friends, he managed to interview Benazir Bhutto at a time when she was not seeing anyone due to an illness. He even sneaked into Karachi Central Jail to interview its most famous prisoner, Asif Ali Zardari, the future president of Pakistan.

Arun also interviewed Prime Minister Nawaz Sharif for *India Today* in the early nineties, during an earlier term of his office. He was pleasantly surprised when Sharif spotted him at the Earth Summit in Rio and came over to shake hands.

He was deeply committed to peace in the subcontinent region. He was clearly concerned about where Pakistan was headed, sharing his Pakistani friends' concerns over the dangers of a policy that promoted and protected jihadis—sadly, a realization that has come rather late to the Pakistani establishment. While he was disturbed about the rise of Hindutva in India, he could not accept that Narendra Modi would one day be the country's Prime Minister, elected by a majority. We often argued when I made this prediction, and I would accuse him of being in denial. Even when Modi won, he believed that Indians had voted against the Congress, rather than *for* Modi. Although Arun had stopped coming to Pakistan and my visits to India were infrequent, India-Pakistan relations were close to his heart and we had long discussions over the phone about our respective countries' slides into intolerance.

On my first visit to Delhi in 1987, Arun not only put me up but acted as a tour guide, obviously taking pleasure in showing me the sights of Delhi, a city he clearly loved. He also made arrangements for me to travel to Agra to see the Taj Mahal. It was on this visit that I got to know his family, his wife Arati and son Adil, who was only ten years old at the time. Years later in 2009, I, along with two other friends from Pakistan, would attend Adil's wedding in Delhi and Samode. I remember how proud Arun was of his son and always remembered to share all the good news about him—jobs, promotions, success at finding a life partner in

Samini. Later, he would take great pleasure in sharing news and pictures of his grandchildren, Arman and Seher.

I last spent time with Arun when I visited him in August 2011. He was already ill but well enough to go out. Later, as his health deteriorated, I made it a point of calling him every Sunday. I could sense his voice getting weaker and later, he would sometimes hand the phone to Arati. I was in a dilemma about visiting him. Part of me wanted to see him for the last time, part of me wanted to retain the memory of a friend as I had last seen him. When I called on June 16, 2015, Arun's voice sounded surprisingly healthy. When I said 'Arun?', Adil handed the phone to his mother, who informed me that Arun had passed away that afternoon.

I.A. Rehman

Rehman Sahib, a leading journalist and human rights activist in Pakistan, was special to Arun—no visit to Pakistan was complete without meeting him. He wrote:

> Although I had the good fortune of knowing Arun Chacko for close to three decades, it was only after his death that I realized that he did not allow me to look deep enough into his life to enable me to paint his complete portrait. But whatever I could learn about him is enough for him to qualify as an absolutely upright person whose friendship any decent human being would have eagerly sought—steeped completely in the finest traditions of secularism.
>
> My friendship with Arun began at our very first meeting, when he walked into the modest office of *Weekly Viewpoint* during the early years of General Zia-ul-Haq's dictatorship. He was prominent in the stream of Indian journalists for whom General Zia rolled out precious carpets (which could often be packed in the home-bound baggage) obviously driven by his craze to be accepted as a benign ruler.
>
> What struck me most was that, unlike quite a few journalists from India, Arun approached the Zia phenomenon with a robust skepticism. He had been taken in neither by Zia's homilies on democracy nor by his overly laboured

humility. He made no secret about his fears for the people of Pakistan, and was keen to find out about the strength of the democratic elements in the country. That, in fact, was the reason for his call at the *Viewpoint*.

He established his credentials as a serious journalist within a few minutes of our meeting. He kept his voice so low that sometimes he was barely audible, phrased his questions carefully, avoided speaking before you had finished your sentence, and chose to wait for the discussion to move towards a definite conclusion.

Arun's qualities as a friend became clear to me when I visited New Delhi in 1987, a little more than 40 years after my last visit to the city in 1947. Arun drove me all over the town in his jeep. He was also generous with his advice about whom to meet for getting an insight into Indian politics, and which of the names on my list deserved to be dropped.

He would often recall his happy childhood days in Gorakhpur where people belonging to different faiths lived together in peace and harmony. His family had extremely happy relations with many families of large-hearted Muslims. In subsequent years, his fears about South Asia's religious bigotry and intolerance pushed him to the brink of despair.

I cannot recall what made Arun drift away from journalism, though his unhappiness over the decline of media barons' standard of probity was no secret. Perhaps, believing in his talent, he accepted the challenge of new media. Many were taken by surprise when Arun suddenly changed course and took up the cause of conservation. The many years he had spent in Switzerland were marked by a single-minded professionalism. It was as a conservation specialist that he once visited Pakistan, and he and I were able to share a few jokes at the expense of the intelligence sleuths who had come to ask me about the arrival date of my friend from India—when he had already gone back.

Soft-spoken and extraordinarily polite most of the time, Arun could surprise his company with a sudden burst of anger when he thought it necessary to put a corrupt politician in his place. He often criticized the South Asian experiments in blocking the people's right to democracy, and wondered how long it would take for the region to produce honest, truthful and conscientious builders of a just society.

I regret that I did not get an opportunity to witness his battle against a deadly affliction, but I can believe the accounts of his courageous bearing in moments of extreme pain—that was a part of his character. His strong will had enabled him to sail through testing times without compromising on his convictions. He won respect without craving it.

Kamran Shafi

Arun had met Kamran Shafi, a fellow journalist, on his innumerable trips to Pakistan. Currently, Kamran Shafi is Pakistan's ambassador to Havana. Kamran Shafi wrote:

> I first met Arun Chacko in Lahore during the height of Zia-ul-Haq's tyranny, and that of the Movement for the Restoration of Democracy (MRD) in the year, if memory serves so many years later, 1983.
>
> He was then writing for *The Indian Express*, before he went on write for other publications. His subject was always politics, whether he was writing on the Emergency in India, and the MRD movement in Pakistan, or the Reykjavik summit between Regan and Gorbachev.
>
> Arun was a friend of friends, and it didn't matter that five or six years passed without contact, and whether we met in India or in Pakistan; his spontaneous warmth made it seem we had met just the week before.
>
> He was a listener, and whilst discussing something would quietly let people finish what they were saying, and then in his gentle way agree or even disagree with a cogent and intelligent argument—making his point in no uncertain terms, but always calmly.
>
> Rest in peace dear friend, who walked gently upon the earth. I miss you.

Anil Kalra

Anil Kalra was a more recent addition to his list of friends, from his days in Switzerland. Anil turned out to be steadfast in his loyalty, visiting at least once in ten days when Arun's health worsened. Anil Kalra wrote:

> It was in the autumn of 1997. I was going on a three-month-long consulting engagement with the United Nations to Geneva. Over dinner, a common friend mentioned Arun Chacko, a schoolmate from Sherwood College, Nainital, currently a Communications Director at the World Wildlife Fund of Nature in Gland, Switzerland. The name rang a bell. I recalled a senior by the same name at the Methodist High School in Kanpur. Too much of a coincidence!
>
> I arrived in Geneva with only Arun's email address. Eager to make contact with the only friendly reference I had, I sent him an introductory email. I also recollected an account of an Arun Chacko at least four years my senior in school—but that reference was merely to highlight the similarity of names!
>
> Within minutes I had a response: 'I am the Chacko who finished school with Vimal Mohindra—and the same Chacko who was at Methodist High School till Class 9.' As it turned out, Arun's father was Professor of Philosophy at Christ Church College, Kanpur (my alma mater), and he had spent his formative years in my hometown. The mail went further, inviting me for dinner the same evening. He lived in Gland, a village about twenty minutes from Geneva.
>
> Over a glass of rather good red wine, the conversation was easy-going and engaging, like that between two long-lost buddies. This was the start of our friendship, an eighteen-year journey with one of the finest, most sincere and true friends that one can ever have.
>
> I learnt a lot from Arun. His knowledge of literature, history, current affairs and international relations was absolutely amazing. He had an insatiable passion for learning and read voraciously. He was quite an encyclopedia

of information and we could spend hours debating and solving the problems of this world!

Arun had an amazing network of friends—be it classmates from his school days in Kanpur or Nainital, or his college network from St Stephen's College in Delhi, or his journalist friends, business associates and professional colleagues. He was never alone, and if there were no friends around he would surround himself with newspapers and books—there was never a dull moment in his life.

On our return to Delhi we continued to remain in touch, often meeting for lunch. His quest for good food remained steadfast, throughout health or sickness. He was always the first person to have tried the newest restaurant in town.

Arun, my mentor and dear friend, I miss you and our banter, which usually started with a greeting—'Sarkaar, kya haal hain?' It was a friendship I cherish, for all the good times we had together.

George Verghese

Dr George Verghese (Reji) was a cousin of sorts, an exemplary human and a complete foodie like Arun—surely it was the genetic link between the two. Reji loved to mother Arun. When we arrived in Boston in January 2013 for his treatment, he had a pair of warm gloves and a woollen scarf ready, bracing him for the cold weather. He was meticulous in what he did—he even taught me to load the washing machine his way. I'm not sure I remember it now—whether it was from right to left or starting from below and going upwards. This is what Reji wrote:

> Arun Chacko and I are cousins. I was born six years after him. My mother and his father are related, though I couldn't explain to you how; they grew up in adjacent towns in Kerala, but may never have met. His father travelled to north India as a young man, and my mother left for (then) Ceylon and subsequently, Ethiopia, and eventually to the US. It fell to Arun, mainly after his father's passing, to seek

out his Kerala roots and knit that branch of the family into his life. I was one beneficiary of this mission. Over the decades since we first met, he became the closest I had to an older brother.

It was on the Madras Christian College (MCC) campus, at the home of a common uncle who was the college doctor, that I first met Arun. I remember being impressed even then by his smart bearing and his polished manner. I was also struck by the way he asked me questions with genuine interest, and listened to my answers more attentively and respectfully than I was used to being listened to in my mid-teens. I had less success at getting him to talk about himself, but I recall later being impressed to learn that he had sailed on a tramp steamer to Basra and beyond when he was just nineteen!

In 1989, Arun had come to our wedding at the Memorial Church on the Stanford University campus. We've also conspired to meet in other Indian cities—Cochin and Bangalore, as well as abroad. But most of our other meetings have been in Boston—both during my bachelor days and regularly afterwards as well, including in his months of treatment here two years before his passing.

Our home in Boston was always his. He was our first houseguest in the place where we have lived now for twenty years. He watched our daughters Deia and Amaya grow up. He had been here with us through the worst of winter. On the morning of 9/11 in 2001, we paced in front of the TV together as the horrors of the day unfolded, and shared our fears of everything that would be unleashed by this catastrophe. He had flown into Boston just the previous day from Dulles airport outside Washington D.C., from where one of the 9/11 planes departed the next day.

We were blessed to have Arun with us during his last extended stay in Boston in 2013, while he underwent treatment at Dana Farber. He had a special connection with Amaya, who has autism. They both enjoyed their daily interactions—she'd smile happily and oblige when Uncle Arun said, 'Drink your milk, baby.' He also enjoyed Ann's cooking, especially the Kerala dishes. He astonished us time and again with his memory of people, events, places and meals from decades earlier. And his analysis of social and political happenings around the world was unfailingly illuminating.

In May 2015, in the week between the end of classes and the final school exams here in Boston, I flew to Delhi and stayed in a hotel near Sainik Farms, spending a good part of each day with Arun. What really perked up Arun's mealtimes was Kerala food from a nearby restaurant. We ordered take-out for a meal, and he set aside the more sensible food that he was dutifully eating at home, in order to tackle the fish curry and avial, along with the other treats on offer. And after one such lunch, we said a tearful goodbye, promising to see each other in some future space-time.

Coda

I was encouraging Amaya with something the other day, and we had the following exchange:
Me: Come on, Amaya, you can do it!
Amaya: Let's show Uncle Arun.
Me: Yes, let's show him. But he's not here, honey.
Amaya: Uncle Arun's sleeping.
Me: Yes, he's sleeping.
Amaya: Uncle Arun loves you.
Me: Yes, sweetie, he loves you.

Rakesh Jayal and Shailendra Pandey

There were many other friends who helped him in his battle against cancer by keeping in constant touch and showing him they were mindful of his ordeal. Some were in contact on an almost daily basis, particularly when the going got tough and he needed them the most. Two people were steadfast in their caring of him—Rakesh Jayal, a friend from his earlier stint with the Press Institute of India, and a school friend—Shailendra Pandey, who never failed to entertain him with his frequent witty telephone calls.

In life, everyone needs a friend like Rakesh. When he was not travelling, he took time out to visit Arun at least five times a week, braving Delhi traffic at peak hours. He provided the diversion Arun needed, and helped keep him connected to the outside world—diminishing the hopelessness of his condition. The progressing cancer was forgotten for those few moments of conversation with Rakesh, taking him to another level, perhaps even happiness.

Arun took his visits for granted, talking about him and looking out for him around six every evening, even when he could not come. Rakesh himself is not a calm person *per se*, but his charm, warmth, and concern had an enormously calming influence on Arun—instantly distracting him from his disease. A discussion about history, the current political scenario or memories from their past kept his mind ticking.

Rakesh visited Arun in the hospital when he developed haematuria, and at a time when he was extremely dejected, depressed and feeling crushed by the hopelessness of his situation. Rakesh was there for his last communion, even though his wife had been admitted to a nearby hospital.

Epilogue

Yesterday I was clever,
So I wanted to change the world.
Today I am wise,
So I am changing myself.

—Rumi

Great strides have been made and continue to be made in the diagnosis and treatment of cancer. Modern medicine adds newer and, potentially, more effective drugs to its arsenal of treatments every year, almost at a breakneck speed, to somehow reduce the mortality from cancer. However, the incidence of the disease continues to climb unrelentingly along with the mortalities from it.

If we give any credence to the claim by the World Cancer Research Fund that most cancers are preventable,[81] then individually each one of us must take on the responsibility of improving our lifestyles. We must be judicious and make considered choices regarding our lives, in addition to being mindful of the dos and donts of a healthy diet. Surely, following some of these basic thumb rules would result in a significant reduction in the rate of this dreaded disease.

Some, even after a courageous fight, will succumb to cancer which has completely taken over their bodies. Others, the more fortunate ones, may somehow manage to restore their health by correcting the imbalances in their bodies—perhaps by strengthening their immune system to fight the scourge from within. These lucky ones may successfully restore their bodies to almost full health by maintaining the vigil. By not falling back into the old ways, what has been achieved can hopefully be secured.

The corrective measures taken must somehow be held on to, to ensure that another similar episode of such immense suffering does not come our way. Paying attention to our bodies, the only possession that is truly ours, is the way forward. In other words, having regained our health we must retain the wellness. Healthy eating implies consuming a balanced diet, i.e. eating in moderation and including a wide spectrum of nutrients.

Diet types and dietary constituents which provide protection during the treatment of cancer, will continue to protect us thereafter—if only we can stick to them. The emphasis should remain on the three important aspects of our lives—diet, weight control and physical activity. Cancer survivors need to follow a healthy diet, keeping in mind the tips for remaining healthy. Choosing nourishing food and drink instead of only dietary supplements is the way to vitality.

Just when the caterpillar thought the world was over,
it became a butterfly.

Life is beautiful. Nobody needs a serious illness to discover this. We can keep our bodies intact and salubrious, and enjoy the life we have. The more we realize its beauty and make whatever little changes needed to achieve good health, the more likely we are to succeed. The ingredients of this success lies in a diet predominantly rich in plant food, high in nutrients and dietary fibre, low in energy-dense foods or non-starchy fruits and vegetables. This affords protection against cancer but also against obesity. Exercise is the other limb of this triangle which improves the equilibrium between our body and our mind.

Fortunately, Indians are largely vegetarian, therefore the changes required to comply with the recommended diets for cancer protection in this book are but a few. There are plenty of effective phytochemicals and protective spices in our foods. However, our diet tends to be starchy, rich in deep-fried food and Indian sweets which are pure sugar. Restricting their intake, or even eliminating some of these would automatically bring greater health into our lives. Considering that we have little individual control on the worsening environmental pollution (though adopting eco-friendly practices such as waste segregation and using renewable energy does make a difference), or the contaminated water supply, we can at least make the right choices with food. All of us can surely determine what we eat.

As India moves towards hyper-industrialization, we shouldn't move away from our healthier, predominantly plant-based diet to a Western diet rich in animal proteins and refined carbohydrates. It is accepted knowledge that lifestyle choices affect the chance of developing cancer.[82] Avoiding all forms of tobacco, eating a plant-rich diet, drinking in moderation, limiting the intake of processed meats, pickles and Indian sweets, eating mixed nuts, maintaining a healthy weight and being active are very germane and straightforward steps.

It may be much harder to determine who will heal us when we are sick. Medical institutions are meant to impart knowledge and skills to their students. Ostensibly, good medical education includes medical ethics and good bedside manners. In a study conducted in 2011 at the two premier medical institutions of north India— AIIMS, New Delhi and PGIMER, Chandigarh, patient dissatisfaction was reported to be at 45 per cent.[83] The patients' feedback indicated low levels of satisfaction with the behaviour of the staff.

Both these institutions were created with the mandate to improve the level and quality of medical education in the country. After their training, doctors from these institutions are supposed to carry their expertise and skills to other medical centres; firstly, to raise the level of medical knowledge in other parts of the country, and secondly, to improve the standard of patient care. If both these premier institutions have themselves been blacklisted for poor patient satisfaction, what message are their alumni likely to carry with them?

Also, nutritional education is not stressed enough in medical schools. The resulting knowledge gap needs to be compensated for by providing each patient with the optimal therapeutic diet for their ailment—whether it is a chronic disease or a type of cancer. Diet should be an integral part of the treatment regimen.

As doctors, we need to take half a step backwards and rediscover narrative medicine, i.e. paying attention to the patient's narrative. The key to narrative medicine lies in listening and heeding to the needs of the patient. In many ways, the importance given to the doctor-patient relationship, in medicine, is progressively diminishing with the disappearance of the family doctor. The doctor-patient relationship should be based on credibility, caring, compassion and sincerity. Instead of focusing on answering questionnaires and doing sophisticated diagnostic procedures and laboratory tests, we need to nurture the art of healing—without ignoring the impact of communication. Each patient has to be treated with profound dignity and respect, regardless of who they are.

Medicine needs to give up its quest for immortality and reconsider the importance of the quality of life. The paradigm of prevention and protection is more conducive to health and well-being—it can bring back the joy in living. For a doctor, it is indeed a privilege that a patient seeks them out for their knowledge and skills, placing their utmost trust into their hands, a trust beyond any other—of life itself. Thus, practising medicine should never, under any circumstance, descend into a money-making scheme, like other businesses.

Acknowledgements

I would like to thank my friends and family for their encouragement, support and constructive criticism during the process of writing this book. Some require special mention: the suggestion to write the book on nutrition during cancer care came from Dr Niraja Gopal Jayal, and I am thankful for her commitment to see it through. I would like to thank Upreet Dhaliwal, Navjeevan Singh, Jayanti and Rakesh Jayal for their advice through the various stages of this book; Royina Grewal, for reading it and helping in finding a publisher; Maya Mirchandani and Ayesha Kapur for their reassurances that helped keep me on track; finally, I am grateful to all the patients who shared their stories with me.

I am also indebted to the contributors of the chapter 'Friends and Remembrances'—Sandy Shaw, Rohit Salve, Zohra Yusuf, I.A. Rehman, Kamran Shafi, Anil Kalra, and George Verghese.

My gratitude to the editors: Shalini Krishan for slowly giving shape to the book and Kartikeya Jain for being a great communicator with immense patience.

References

Facts About Cancer

1. William A. Meissner and George T. Diamandopoulos, "Neoplasia," in *Pathology*, ed. William A. Anderson and John M. Kissane (St. Louis: Mosby, 1977), 640.
2. Ibid.
3. Song Wu, Scott Powers, Wei Zhu and Yusuf A. Hannun, "Substantial Contribution of Extrinsic Risk Factors to Cancer Development," *Nature* 529 (2016): 43-47.
4. Preetha Anand, Ajaikumar B. Kunnumakara, Chitra Sundaram, Kuzhuvelil B. Harikumar, Sheeja T. Tharakan, Oiki S. Lai, Bokyung Sung and Bharat B. Aggarwal, "Cancer Is a Preventable Disease that Requires Major Lifestyle Changes," *Pharmaceutical Research* 25, no. 9 (2008): 2097-2116.

Diagnosis of Cancer

5. Daisuke Ichikawa, Naoya Hashimoto, Masakazu Hoshima, Toshiharu Yamaguchi, Kiyoshi Sawai, Yusuke Nakamura, Toshio Takahashi, Tatsuo Abe and Johji Inazawa, "Analysis of Numerical Aberrations in Specific Chromosomes by Fluorescent In Situ Hybridization as a Diagnostic Tool in Breast Cancer," *Cancer* 77 (1996), 2064-69.

Grappling with the Diagnosis

6. Maggie K. Hughes, "The Role of Support Groups in Cancer Survivorship," *Advancing Your Health* (blog), May 17, 2012, 3:06 pm, http://advancingyourhealth.org/cancer/2012/05/17/cancer-support-groups-survivorship/.

Quality of Life

7. World Health Organization, "WHOQOL: Measuring Quality of Life," accessed on July 12, 2018. http://www.who.int/healthinfo/survey/whoqol-qualityoflife/en/.
8. Gregory Garra, Adam J. Singer, Anna Domingo and Henry C.

Thode, "The Wong-Baker Pain FACES Scale Measures Pain, Not Fear," *Pediatric Emergency Care* 29, no. 1 (2013): 17–20.

9. Marcia Testa and Donal Simonson, "Assessment of Quality of Life Outcomes," *The New England Journal of Medicine* 334, no. 13 (1996): 835–840.
10. Neil K. Aaronson, Sam Ahmedzai, Bengt Bergman, Monika Bullinger, Ann Cull, Nicole J. Duez, Antonio J. Filiberti, Henning Flechtner, Stewart B. Fleishman, Johanna C.J.M. de Haes, Stein Kaasa, Marianne Klee, David Osoba, Darius Razavi, Peter B. Rofe, Simon Schraub, Kommer Sneeuw, Marianne Sullivan and Fumikazu Takeda, "A Quality-Of-Life Instrument for Use in International Clinical Trials in Oncology," *JNCI: Journal of the National Cancer Institute* 85, no. 5 (1993): 365-376.

Why Did Cancer Develop?

11. Bernard W. Stewart and C.P. Wild, eds. *World Cancer Report 2014* (Geneva: World Health Organisation, 2014), 124-303.
12. "2018 WHO ranking of polluted cities explained, bad news for India," CSE India. Last modified May 10, 2018, https://www.cseindia.org/2018-who-ranking-of-polluted-cities-explainced-bad-news-for-india-8673.

Cancer Treatments

13. "Cell cycle," Wikipedia. Last modified October 8, 2018, https://en.wikipedia.org/wiki/Cell_cycle.

Drug Resistance

14. Alessandro Torgovnick and Björn Schumacher, "DNA Repair Mechanisms in Cancer Development and Therapy," *Frontiers in Genetics* 6 (2015): 157.

The Relationship Between Food and Cancer

15. Preetha Anand, et al., "Cancer is a Preventable Disease that Requires Major Lifestyle Changes," *Pharmaceutical Research* 25, no. 9 (2008): 2097-2116.
16. "UN General Assembly proclaims Decade of Action on

Nutrition," Food and Agriculture Organization of the United Nations. Last modified July 30, 2017, http://www.fao.org/news/story/en/item/408970/icode/.

17. Carlos A. Monteiro, Geoffrey Cannon, Renata Levy, Jean-Claude Moubarac, Patricia Jaime, Ana Paula Martins, Daniela Canella, Maria Louzada and Diana Parra, "NOVA: The Star Shines Bright," *World Nutrition* 7, no. 1-3 (2016), 28-38.
18. Thibault Fiolet, Laury Sellem, Benjamin Allès, Mélanie Deschasaux, Philippine Fassier, Paule Latino-Martel, Serge Hercberg, Céline Lavalette, Chantal Julia and Mathilde Touvier, "Consumption of Ultra-Processed Foods and Cancer Risk: Results from NutriNet-Santé Prospective Cohort," last modified September 24, 2018, https://www.bmj.com/content/360/bmj.k322.
19. Carlos A. Monteiro, Geoffrey Cannon, Renata Levy, et al., "NOVA: The Star Shines Bright," *World Nutrition* 7, no. 1-3 (2016), 28-38.
20. William Haenszel and Minoru Kurihara, "Studies of Japanese Immigrants: Mortality from Cancer and Other Diseases Among Japanese in the United States," *Journal of the National Cancer Institute* 40, no. 1 (1968): 43-68.
21. Suzanne E. Geerlings, and Andy I.M. Hoepelman, "Immune dysfunction in patients with diabetes mellitus (DM)," *FEMS Immunology & Medical Microbiology* 26, no. 3-4 (1999): 259-265.
22. Paula Jakszyn and Carlos Alberto González, "Nitrosamine and Related Food Intake and Gastric and Oesophageal Cancer Risk: A Systematic Review of the Epidemiological Evidence," *World Journal of Gastroenterology* 12, no. 27 (2006): 4296.
23. Mark E. Whalon and Byron A. Wingerd, "Bt: Mode of Action and Use," *Archives of Insect Biochemistry and Physiology: Published in Collaboration with the Entomological Society of America* 54, no. 4 (2003): 200-211.
24. Harris R. Lieberman, Benjamin Caballero, Gail G. Emde and Jerrold G. Bernstein, "The Effects of Aspartame on Human Mood, Performance, and Plasma Amino Acid Levels," in *Dietary Phenylalanine and Brain Function* ed. R. J. Wurtman & E. Ritter-Walker (Boston: Birkhauser, 1988), 198-200.

25. Cristina Bosetti, Silvano Gallus, Renato Talamini, Maurizio Montella, Silvia Franceschi, Eva Negri and Carlo La Vecchia, "Artificial Sweeteners and the Risk of Gastric, Pancreatic, and Endometrial Cancers in Italy," *Cancer Epidemiology and Prevention Biomarkers* 18, no. 8 (2009): 2235–8.
26. Gabriele Amersbach, "The Problem with Emulsifiers: Part 2," accessed on June 21, 2017. https://www.prebiotin.com/the-problem-with-emulsifiers-part-2/.
27. World Health Organization, and Management of Substance Abuse Unit, *Global Status Report on Alcohol and Health, 2014* (Geneva: World Health Organization, 2014).
28. David E. Nelson, Dwayne W. Jarman, Jürgen Rehm, Thomas K. Greenfield, Grégoire Rey, William C. Kerr, Paige Miller, Kevin D. Shield, Yu Ye, and Timothy S. Naimi, "Alcohol-Attributable Cancer Deaths and Years of Potential Life Lost in the United States," *American Journal of Public Health* 103, no. 4 (2013): 641-648.
29. Nathalie M. Delzenne and Patrice D. Cani, "A Place for Dietary Fibre in the Management of the Metabolic Syndrome," *Current Opinion in Clinical Nutrition & Metabolic Care* 8, no. 6 (2005): 636–640.
30. Eleonora Ciarlo, Tytti Heinonen, Jacobus Herderschee, Craig Fenwick, Matteo Mombelli, Didier Le Roy and Thierry Roger, "Impact of Microbial Derived Short Chain Fatty Acid Propionate on Host Susceptibility to Bacterial and Fungal Infections in Vivo," *Scientific Reports* 6 (2016): 37944.
31. Peter H. Gann, Robert T. Chatterton, Susan M. Gapstur, Kiang Liu, Daniel Garside, Sue Giovanazzi, Kim Thedford and Linda Van Horn, "The Effects of a Low-Fat/High-Fiber Diet on Sex Hormone Levels and Menstrual Cycling in Premenopausal Women: A 12-Month Randomized Trial (the Diet and Hormone Study)," *Cancer* 98, no. 9 (2003): 1870.
32. In addition, there was weight loss. Weight control may therefore be considered a feasible approach in lowering the levels of female hormones in the body by reducing the total body fat.
33. Susanna C. Larsson, Niclas Håkansson, Edward Giovannucci and Alicja Wolk, "Folate Intake and Pancreatic Cancer

Incidence: A Prospective Study of Swedish Women and Men," *Journal of the National Cancer Institute* 98, no. 6 (2006): 407.
34. Joan M. Lappe, Dianne Travers-Gustafson, K. Michael Davies, Robert R. Recker and Robert P. Heaney, "Vitamin D and Calcium Supplements Reduce Cancer Risk: Results of a Randomized Trial," *The American Journal of Clinical Nutrition* 85, no. 6 (2007): 1586.
35. Kathleen Y. Wolin, Kenneth Carson and Graham A. Colditz, "Obesity and Cancer," *The Oncologist* 15, no. 6 (2010): 556-565.
36. Andrew G. Renehan, Margaret Tyson, Matthias Egger, Richard F. Heller and Marcel Zwahlen, "The Body Mass Index: A Systematic Review and Meta-Analysis of Prospective Observational Study," *The Lancet* 371, no. 9612 (2008): 569.
37. Gillian K. Reeves, Kirstin Pirie, Valerie Beral, Jane Green, Elizabeth Spencer and Diana Bull, "Cancer Incidence and Mortality in Relation to Body Mass Index in the Million Women Study: Cohort Study," *BMJ* 335, no. 7630 (2007): 1134.
38. Hutan Ashrafian, Kamran Ahmed, Simon P. Rowland, Vanash M. Patel, Nigel J. Gooderham, Elaine Holmes, Ara Darzi, and Thanos Athanasiou, "Metabolic Surgery and Cancer: Protective Effects of Bariatric Procedures," *Cancer* 117, no. 9 (2011): 1788-89.
39. Ibid.
40. World Cancer Research Fund and American Institute for Cancer Research, *Continuous Update Project Expert Report 2018* (London: World Cancer Research Fund, 2018), 15-33.

Using the Beneficial Effects of Food in Cancer

41. K Lawrence H. Kushi, Colleen Doyle, Marji McCullough, Cheryl L. Rock, Wendy Demark-Wahnefried, Elisa V. Bandera, Susan Gapstur, Alpa V. Patel, Kimberly Andrews, Ted Gansler and The American Cancer Society 2010 Nutrition and Physical Activity Guidelines Advisory Committee, "American Cancer Society Guidelines on Nutrition and Physical Activity for Cancer Prevention: Reducing the Risk of Cancer with Healthy Food Choices and Physical Activity," *CA: A Cancer Journal for Clinicians* 62, no. 1 (2012): 30-67.

42. Ibid.
43. Fergus Walsh, "How exercise in old age prevents the immune system from declining," last modified June 23, 2018. http://www.bbc.com/news/health-43308729.
44. World Federation for Mental Health, *Depression: A Global Crisis* (Occoquan: World Federation for Mental Health, 2012), 6. www.who.int/mental_health/.../depression/wfmh_paper_depression_wmhd_2012.pdf.
45. Barbara L. Andersen, William B. Farrar, Deanna Golden-Kreutz, Leigh Ann Kutz, Robert MacCallum, Mary Elizabeth Courtney, and Ronald Glaser, "Stress and Immune Responses after Surgical Treatment Of Regional Breast Cancer," *JNCI: Journal of the National Cancer Institute* 90, no. 1 (1998): 30.
46. Susan K. Lutgendorf, Anil K. Sood, Barrie Anderson, Stephanie McGinn, Heena Maiseri, Minh Dao, Joel I. Sorosky, Koen De Geest, Justine Ritchie, and David M. Lubaroff, "Social Support, Psychological Distress and Natural Killer Cell Activity In Ovarian Cancer," *Journal of Clinical Oncology* 23, no. 28 (2005): 7105.
47. Linda C. Nebeling, Floro Miraldi, S. B. Shurin, and E. Lerner, "Effects of a Ketogenic Diet on Tumour Metabolism and Nutritional Status in Pediatric Oncology Patients: Two Case Reports," *Journal of the American College of Nutrition* 14, no. 2 (1995): 202.
48. GB Health Watch, "Omega-3 : Omega-6 balance," accessed October 27, 2017. https://www.gbhealthwatch.com/Science-Omega3-Omega6.php.
49. Anne C. Thiébaut, Véronique Chajès, Mariette Gerber, Marie-Christine Boutron-Ruault, Virginie Joulin, Gilbert Lenoir, Franco Berrino, Elio Riboli, Jacques Bénichou, and Françoise Clavel-Chapelon, "Dietary Intakes of Omega-6 and Omega-3 Polyunsaturated Fatty Acids and the Risk of Breast Cancer," *International Journal of Cancer* 124, no. 4 (2009): 924-931.
50. World Cancer Research Fund and American Institute for Cancer Research, *Food, Nutrition, Physical Activity, and the Prevention of Cancer: A Global Perspective* (Washington DC: American Institute for Cancer Research, 2007).
51. Bharat B. Aggarwal, Chitra Sundaram, Nikita Malani, and

Haruyo Ichikawa, "Curcumin: The Indian Solid Gold," in *The Molecular Targets and Therapeutic Uses of Curcumin In Health And Disease* (Boston: Springer, 2007), 11-12.

52. Bharat B. Aggarwal, Haruyo Ichikawa, Prachi Garodia, Priya Weerasinghe, Gautam Sethi, Indra D. Bhatt, Manoj K. Pandey, Shishir Shishodia, and Muraleedharan G. Nair, "The Traditional Ayurvedic Medicine to Modern Medicine: Identification of Therapeutic Targets for Suppression of Inflammation and Cancer," *Expert Opinion on Therapeutic Targets* 10, no. 1 (2006): 87-118.
53. Joanna L. Slavin, "Mechanisms for the Impact of Whole Grain Food on Cancer Risk," *Journal of the American College of Nutrition* 19, no. 3 (2000): 300S-307S.
54. Seema Patel and Arun Goyal, "Recent Development in Mushroom as Anti-Cancer Therapeutics: A Review," *Biotech* 3, no. 1 (2012): 1-15.
55. Lélia Figueiredo, "Medicinal Mushroom in Adjuvant Cancer Therapy: An Approach to Anti-Cancer Effect and Presumed Action," *Nutrire* 42, no. 1 (2017): 28.
56. Ibid.
57. World Health Organization, *2008–2013 Action Plan for the Global Strategy for the Prevention and Control of Non-Communicable Diseases* (Geneva: WHO Press, 2008).
58. Myung-Hee Shin, Michelle D. Holmes, Susan E. Hankinson, Kana Wu, Graham A. Colditz, and Walter C. Willett, "Intake of Dairy Products, Calcium, and Vitamin D And Risk of Breast Cancer," *Journal of the National Cancer Institute* 94, no. 17 (2002): 1301.
59. Ibid.
60. "8 Surprising Health Benefits of Cloves," *Healthline*, accessed on 13 October, 2017. https://www.healthline.com/nutrition/benefits-of-cloves.
61. Campos Vega, B. Rocio, Dave Oomah, Guadalupe Loarca-Piña, and Haydé Azeneth Vergara-Castañeda, "Common Beans and their Non-Digestible Faction: Cancer Inhibitory Activity—An Overview," *Foods* 2, no. 3 (2013): 374.
62. Leena Hilakivi-Clarke, Juan E. Andrade, and William Helferich, "Is Soy Consumption Good or Bad for Breast Cancer?" *The Journal of Nutrition* 140, no. 12 (2010): 23265.

63. Mindy Kurzer, "Hormonal Effects of Soy Isoflavones: Studies in Premenopausal and Postmenopausal Women," *The Journal of Nutrition* 130, no. 3 (2000): 660S–661S.
64. Erin L. Richman, Peter R. Carroll, and June M. Chan, "Vegetable and Fruit Intake after Diagnosis and Risk of Prostate Cancer Progression," *International Journal of Cancer* 131, no. 1 (2012): 201.
65. Kristi Steinmetz, Lawrence H. Kushi, Roberd M. Bostick, Aaron R. Folsom, and John D. Potter, "Vegetables, Fruit, and Colon Cancer in the Iowa Women's Health Study," *Rehabilitation Oncology* 112, no. 2 (1994): 19.
66. Hong-Mei Zhang, Lei Zhao, Hao Li, Hao Xu, Wen-Wen Chen, and Lin Tao, "Research Progress on the Anti-carcinogenic Actions and Mechanisms of Ellagic Acid," *Cancer Biology and Medicine* 11, no. 2 (2014): 92–100.

Surgery and Nutrition

67. Savitri Bhatia, *Savitri Bhatia's Culinary Legacy*, ed. Arati Bhatia (New Delhi: Vij Publications, 2016), 114-16.

Chemotherapy and Nutrition

68. See *Savitri Bhatia's Culinary Legacy* (2016).

Managing Palliative Care

69. WHO Expert Committee, *Cancer Pain Relief and Palliative Care* (Geneva: World Health Organization, 1990): 1-75.
70. Marie Bakitas, Tor D. Tosteson, Zhigang Li, Kathleen D. Lyons, Jay G. Hull, Zhongze Li, J. Nicholas Dionne-Odom, Jennifer Frost, Konstantin H. Dragnev, Mark T. Hegel, Andres Azuero, and Tim A. Ahles, "Early Versus Delayed Initiation of Concurrent Palliative Care: Patient Outcomes in the ENABLE III Randomized Controlled Trial," *Journal of Clinical Oncology* 33, no. 13 (2015): 1438.
71. Joseph Greer, William F. Pirl, Vicki A. Jackson, Alona Muzikansky, Inga T. Lennes, Emily R. Gallagher, Holly G. Prigerson, and Jennifer S. Temel, "Perception of Health Status and Survival In Patients With Metastatic Lung Cancer,"

Journal of Pain and Symptom Management 48, no. 4 (2014): 548-557.

72. J. Nicholas Dionne-Odom, Andres Azuero, Kathleen D. Lyons, Jay G. Hull, Tor Tosteson, Zhigang Li, Zhongze Li, Jennifer Frost, Konstantin H. Dragnev, Imatullah Akyar, Mark T. Hegel, and Marie A. Bakitas, "Benefits of Early Versus Delayed Palliative Care to Informal Family Caregivers of Patients with Advanced Cancer: Outcomes from ENABLE III Randomized Controlled Trial," *Journal of Clinical Oncology* 33, no. 13 (2015): 1446-1452.
73. "WHO's cancer pain ladder for adults," World Health Organization, accessed on August 13, 2017. www.who.int/cancer/palliative/painladder/en/.

Diagnosis and Starting Treatment

74. Sarah Belle Dougherty, "Music and the Healing Arts," accessed on 21 June, 2018. http://www.theosophy-nw.org/theosnw/death/he-sbd.htm.

The Sense of Touch

75. Joseph Stromberg, "9 surprising facts about the sense of touch," Vox, Jan 28, 2015. https://www.vox.com/2015/1/28/7925737/touch-facts.
76. Adam Gopnik, "Feel Me," *The New Yorker*, accessed on May 13, 2017. https://www.newyorker.com/magazine/2016/05/16/what-the-science-of-touch-says-about-us.

Discussions About Life and Death

77. "The State of Euthanasia In Europe," accessed on January 4, 2018. https://medicalxpress.com/news/2014-12-state-euthanasia-europe.html.
78. "Death with Dignity Act," accessed on January 4, 2018. https://www.oregon.gov/oha/PH/PROVIDERPARTNERRESOURCES/EVALUATIONRESEARCH/DEATHWITHDIGNITYACT/Pages/index.aspx.
79. "Social interaction can help cancer patients survive longer," *QCityMetro*, accessed on October 13, 2018. https://qcitymetro.

com/2017/07/24/social-interaction-helps-cancer-patients-survive/.

80. "Passive euthanasia allowed: Read full text of Supreme Court judgment recognising right to die with dignity," FirstPost, accessed on May 9, 2018. https://www.firstpost.com/india/passive-euthanasia-allowed-read-full-text-of-supreme-court-judgment-recognising-right-to-die-with-dignity-4383531.html.

Epilogue

81. World Cancer Research Fund and American Institute for Cancer Research, *Food, Nutrition, Physical Activity, and the Prevention of Cancer: A Global Perspective* (Washington DC: American Institute for Cancer Research, 2007).
82. Naghma Khan, Farrukh Afaq, and Hasan Mukhtar, "Lifestyle as risk factor for cancer: Evidence from human studies," *Cancer Letters* 293, no. 2 (2010): 133-143.
83. Raman Sharma, Meenakshi Sharma, and R. K. Sharma. "The patient satisfaction study in a multispecialty tertiary level hospital, PGIMER, Chandigarh, India." *Leadership in Health Services* 24, no. 1 (2011): 64-73.

Further Reading

Adolfsson, Oskar, Simin Nikbin Meydani, and Robert M. Russell. "Yogurt and gut function." *The American Journal of Clinical Nutrition* 80, no. 2 (2004): 245-256.

Ali, Shahin Sharif, Naresh Kasoju, Abhinav Luthra, Angad Singh, Hallihosur Sharanabasava, Abhishek Sahu, and Utpal Bora. "Indian Medicinal Herbs as Sources of Antioxidants." *Food Research International* 41, no. 1 (2008): 1-15.

Almeida, L. F., and T. Machado Coimbra. "Vitamin D actions on cell differentiation, proliferation and inflammation." *International Journal on Complementary & Alternative Medicine* 6, no. 5 (2017): 00201.

Alfarouk, Khalid O., Christian-Martin Stock, Sophie Taylor, Megan Walsh, Abdel Khalig Muddathir, Daniel Verduzco, Adil H.H. Bashir, Osama Y. Mohammed, Gamal O. Elhassan, Salvador Harguindey, Stephan J. Reshkin, Muntaser E. Ibrahim and Cyril Rauch. "Resistance to Cancer Chemotherapy: Failure in Drug Response from ADME to P-gp." *Cancer Cell International* 15, no. 1 (2015): 71.

Alpert, M. E., R. Hutt, G. N. Wogan, and C. S. Davidson. "Association between aflatoxin content of food and hepatoma frequency in Uganda." *Cancer* 28, no. 1 (1971): 253-260.

Weihrauch, M. R., and V. Diehl. "Artificial sweeteners—do they bear a carcinogenic risk?." *Annals of Oncology* 15, no. 10 (2004): 1460-1465.

Bakitas, Marie, Kathleen Doyle Lyons, Mark T. Hegel, Stefan Balan, Frances C. Brokaw, Janette Seville, Jay G. Hull Zhongze Li, MS; Tor D. Tosteson, ScD; Ira R. Byock, MD; Tim A. Ahles. "Effects of a palliative care intervention on clinical outcomes in patients with advanced cancer: the Project ENABLE II randomized controlled trial." *Jama* 302, no. 7 (2009): 741-749.

Ballard-Barbash, Rachel, David Berrigan, Nancy Potischman, and Emily Dowling. "Obesity and cancer epidemiology." In *Cancer and Energy Balance, Epidemiology and Overview*, edited by Nathan A. Berger, 1-44. New York: Springer, 2010.

Barnard, N. *Foods That Fight Pain*. New York: Harmony Books, 1998.

Baylock, R.L. *Excitotoxins: The Taste That Kills*. Santa Fe: Health Press. 1994.

Bhatia, Arati. "A humbling experience with cancer and chemotherapy." *Medical Humanities* (blog), May 10, 2011, http://blogs.bmj.com/medical-humanities/2011; May.

Bhatia, Arati. "Doctors good and bad." *RHiME* 5 (2018): 20-24.

Blusztajn, J.K. "Choline a vital amine." *Science* 281 (1998): 794.

Bond, C.A., and R. Monson. "Sustained improvement in drug documentation, compliance, and disease control: a four-year analysis of an ambulatory care model." *Archives of Internal Medicine* 144, no. 6 (1984): 1159-62.

Bordia, A., S. K. Verma, and K. C. Srivastava. "Effect of ginger (Zingiber officinale Rosc.) and fenugreek (Trigonella foenumgraecum L.) on blood lipids, blood sugar and platelet aggregation in patients with coronary artery disease." *Prostaglandins, Leukotrienes and Essential Fatty Acids* 56, no. 5 (1997): 379-384.

Boyera, N., I. Galey, and B. A. Bernard. "Effect of vitamin C and its derivatives on collagen synthesis and cross-linking by normal human fibroblasts." *International Journal of Cosmetic Science* 20, no. 3 (1998): 151-158.

Cabrera, Carmen, Reyes Artacho, and Rafael Giménez. "Beneficial effects of green tea—a review." *Journal of the American College of Nutrition* 25, no. 2 (2006): 79-99.

Cabrera, Carmen, Rafael Giménez, and M. Carmen López. "Determination of tea components with antioxidant activity." *Journal of Agricultural and Food Chemistry* 51, no. 15 (2003): 4427-4435.

Calder, Philip C. "Fatty acids and inflammation: the cutting edge between food and pharma." *European Journal of Pharmacology* 668 (2011): S50-S58.

Calder, Philip C. "N–3 Polyunsaturated fatty acids and inflammation: from molecular biology to the clinic." *Lipids* 38, no. 4 (2003): 343-352.

Cartwright, Laura A., Levent Dumenci, Laura A. Siminoff, and Robin K. Matsuyama. "Cancer patients' understanding of prognostic information." *Journal of Cancer Education* 29, no. 2 (2014): 311-317.

Ciarlo, Eleonora, Tytti Heinonen, Jacobus Herderschee, Craig Fenwick, Matteo Mombelli, Didier Le Roy, and Thierry Roger. "Impact of the microbial derived short chain fatty acid propionate on host susceptibility to bacterial and fungal infections in vivo." *Scientific Reports* 6 (2016): 37944.

Hilakivi-Clarke, Leena, Juan E. Andrade, and William Helferich. "Is Soy Consumption Good or Bad for the Breast?." *The Journal of Nutrition* 140, no. 12 (2010): 2326S-2334S.

Constine, L. S., M. T. Milano, and D. Friedman. "Late effects of cancer treatment on normal tissues." In *Principles and Practices of Radiation Oncology*, edited by Halperin, Edward C., Luther W. Brady, Carlos A. Perez, and David E. Wazer, 320. Philadelphia: Lippincott Williams & Wilkins, 2008.

Dancey, J., and S. Arbuck. "Cancer drugs and cancer drug development for the new millennium." In *Progress in Anti-Cancer Chemotherapy*, 91-109. Paris: Springer, 2000.

Danzo, Benjamin J. "Environmental xenobiotics may disrupt normal endocrine function by interfering with the binding of physiological ligands to steroid receptors and binding proteins." *Environmental Health Perspectives* 105, no. 3 (1997): 294.

Dashwood, Roderick, Shane Yamane, and Randy Larsen. "Study of the forces stabilizing complexes between chlorophylls and heterocyclic amine mutagens." *Environmental and Molecular Mutagenesis* 27, no. 3 (1996): 211-218.

de Lorgeril, Michel, and Patricia Salen. "Helping women to good health: breast cancer, omega-3/omega-6 lipids, and related lifestyle factors." *BMC Medicine* 12, no. 1 (2014): 54.

———"New insights into the health effects of dietary saturates and omega-6 and omega-3 polyunsaturated fatty acids." *BMC Medicine* 10, no. 1 (2012): 50.

Dees, Craig, Minoo Askari, James S. Foster, Shamila Ahamed, and Jay Wimalasena. "DDT mimicks estradiol stimulation of breast cancer cells to enter the cell cycle." *Molecular Carcinogenesis: Published in cooperation with the University of Texas MD Anderson Cancer Center* 18, no. 2 (1997): 107-114.

Eldridge, Barbara, and Kathryn K. Hamilton. *Management of Nutrition Impact Symptoms in Cancer and Educational Handouts*. Oncology Nutrition Dietetic Practice Group, American Dietetic Association, 2004.

"Eating hints before, during and after cancer." accessed on May 20, 2015. https://www.cancer.gov/publications/patient-education/eatinghints.pdf.

El-Mallakh, R. S., and M. E. Paskitti. "The ketogenic diet may have mood-stabilizing properties." *Medical Hypotheses* 57, no. 6 (2001): 724-726.

Erickson, Kirk I., Regina L. Leckie, and Andrea M. Weinstein. "Physical activity, fitness, and gray matter volume." *Neurobiology of Aging* 35 (2014): S20-S28.

Ewings, P., and C. Bowie. "A case-control study of cancer of the prostate in Somerset and east Devon." *British Journal of Cancer* 74, no. 4 (1996): 661.

Ferlay, Jacques. "Cancer incidence, mortality and prevalence worldwide." Lyon: IARC Press, 2000.

Fitch, Cindy, and Kathryn S. Keim. "Position of the Academy of Nutrition and Dietetics: use of nutritive and nonnutritive sweeteners." *Journal of the Academy of Nutrition and Dietetics* 112, no. 5 (2012): 739-758.

Freeman, Vincent L., Mohsen Meydani, Kwan Hur, and Robert C. Flanigan. "Inverse association between prostatic polyunsaturated fatty acid and risk of locally advanced prostate carcinoma." *Cancer: Interdisciplinary International Journal of the American Cancer Society* 101, no. 12 (2004): 2744-2754.

Galisteo, Milagros, Juan Duarte, and Antonio Zarzuelo. "Effects of dietary fibers on disturbances clustered in the metabolic syndrome." *The Journal of Nutritional Biochemistry* 19, no. 2 (2008): 71-84.

Gann, Peter H., Robert T. Chatterton, Susan M. Gapstur, Kiang Liu, Daniel Garside, Sue Giovanazzi, Kim Thedford, and Linda

Van Horn. "The effects of a low-fat/high-fiber diet on sex hormone levels and menstrual cycling in premenopausal women: a 12-month randomized trial (the diet and hormone study)." *Cancer* 98, no. 9 (2003): 1870-1879.

Glaser, Adam W., Lorna K. Fraser, Jessica Corner, Richard Feltbower, Eva JA Morris, Greg Hartwell, and Mike Richards. "Patient-reported outcomes of cancer survivors in England 1–5 years after diagnosis: a cross-sectional survey." *BMJ Open* 3, no. 4 (2013): e002317.

Gospodarowicz, Mary K., Brian O'Sullivan, and Leslie H. Sobin, eds. *Prognostic Factors in Cancer*. New York: Wiley-Liss, 2006.

Gosselin-Acomb, T. K. "Principles of radiation therapy." In *Cancer Nursing Principles and Practice*, 229-249. Boston: Jones and Bartlett Publishers, 2005.

Gottesman, Michael M. "Mechanisms of cancer drug resistance." *Annual Review of Medicine* 53, no. 1 (2002): 615-627.

Smith, J. L., S. A. S. Gropper, and J. L. Groff. *Advanced Nutrition and Human Metabolism*. Belmont: Wadsworth Cengage Learning (2009).

Grothey, A., W. Voigt, C. Schöber, T. Müller, W. Dempke, and H. J. Schmoll. "The role of insulin-like growth factor I and its receptor in cell growth, transformation, apoptosis, and chemoresistance in solid tumors." *Journal of Cancer Research and Clinical Oncology* 125, no. 3-4 (1999): 166-173.

Guiney, Hayley, and Liana Machado. "Benefits of regular aerobic exercise for executive functioning in healthy populations." *Psychonomic Bulletin & Review* 20, no. 1 (2013): 73-86.

Halperin, Edward C. "Particle therapy and treatment of cancer." *The Lancet Oncology* 7, no. 8 (2006): 676-685.

Handler, Judd. "Are the benefits of wheat grass overblown?." Mother Nature Network, accessed on November 23, 2015. https://www.mnn.com/health/fitness-well-being/stories/are-the-benefits-of-wheatgrass-overblown.

Hartman, Philip E., and Delbert M. Shankel. "Antimutagens and anticarcinogens: a survey of putative interceptor molecules."

Environmental and Molecular Mutagenesis 15, no. 3 (1990): 145-182.

Hebert, James R., Thomas G. Hurley, Barbara C. Olendzki, Jane Teas, Yunsheng Ma, and Jeffrey S. Hampl. "Nutritional and socioeconomic factors in relation to prostate cancer mortality: a cross-national study." *Journal of the National Cancer Institute* 90, no. 21 (1998): 1637-1647.

Henry, Sara Hale, F. Xavier Bosch, Terry C. Troxell, and P. Michael Bolger. "Reducing liver cancer—global control of aflatoxin." *Science* 286, no. 5449 (1999): 2453-2454.

Hijova, Emilia, and Anna Chmelarova. "Short chain fatty acids and colonic health." *Bratislavské lekárske listy* 108, no. 8 (2007): 354.

Housman, Genevieve, Shannon Byler, Sarah Heerboth, Karolina Lapinska, Mckenna Longacre, Nicole Snyder, and Sibaji Sarkar. "Drug resistance in cancer: an overview." *Cancers* 6, no. 3 (2014): 1769-1792.

Hunter, J. Edward. "n-3 fatty acids from vegetable oils." *The American journal of clinical nutrition* 51, no. 5 (1990): 809-814.

Harbige, Laurence S. "Fatty acids, the immune response, and autoimmunity: a question of n–6 essentiality and the balance between n–6 and n–3." *Lipids* 38, no. 4 (2003): 323-341.

Huston, David P. "The biology of the immune system." *Jama* 278, no. 22 (1997): 1804-1814.

Inserra, Paula F., Sussan K. Ardestani, and Ronald Ross Watson. "Antioxidants and Immune Function." In *Antioxidants and Disease Prevention*, edited by Harinder Garewal, 19-29. New York: CRC Press, 1997.

Jacobsen, Paul B., and Heather S. Jim. "Psychosocial Interventions for Anxiety and Depression in Adult Cancer Patients: Achievements and Challenges." *CA: A Cancer Journal for Clinicians* 58, no. 4 (2008): 214-230.

Kanda, Junya, Keitaro Matsuo, Takeshi Suzuki, Takakazu Kawase, Akio Hiraki, Miki Watanabe, Nobumasa Mizuno, Akira Sawaki, Kenji Yamao, Kazuo Tajima and Hideo Tanaka. "Impact of alcohol consumption with polymorphisms in alcohol-metabolizing enzymes on pancreatic cancer risk in Japanese." *Cancer Science* 100, no. 2 (2009): 296-302.

Kaplan, Jonathan E., Debra Hanson, Mark S. Dworkin, Toni Frederick, Jeanne Bertolli, Mary Lou Lindegren, Scott Holmberg, and Jeffrey L. Jones. "Epidemiology of human immunodeficiency virus-associated opportunistic infections in the United States in the era of highly active antiretroviral therapy." *Clinical Infectious Diseases* 30, no. 1 (2000): S5-S14.

Kelley, Darshan S., and Adnianne Bendich. "Essential nutrients and immunologic functions." *The American Journal of Clinical Nutrition* 63, no. 6 (1996): 994S-996S.

Koenig, Harold, Dana King, and Verna B. Carson. *Handbook of Religion and Health*. New York: Oxford University Press, 2001.

Koury, Mark J., and Prem Ponka. "New insights into erythropoiesis: the roles of folate, vitamin B12, and iron." *Annual Review of Nutrition* 24 (2004): 105-131.

Kry, Stephen F., Mohammad Salehpour, David S. Followill, Marilyn Stovall, Deborah A. Kuban, R. Allen White, and Isaac I. Rosen. "The calculated risk of fatal secondary malignancies from intensity-modulated radiation therapy." *International Journal of Radiation Oncology, Biology, Physics* 62, no. 4 (2005): 1195-1203.

Lambeth, J. David. "NOX enzymes and the biology of reactive oxygen." *Nature Reviews Immunology* 4, no. 3 (2004): 181.

Lappe, Joan M., Dianne Travers-Gustafson, K. Michael Davies, Robert R. Recker, and Robert P. Heaney. "Vitamin D and calcium supplementation reduces cancer risk: results of a randomized trial." *The American Journal of Clinical Nutrition* 85, no. 6 (2007): 1586-1591.

Le, Hien T., Charlene M. Schaldach, Gary L. Firestone, and Leonard F. Bjeldanes. "Plant derived 3, 3'-diindolylmethane is a strong androgen antagonist in human prostate cancer cells." *Journal of Biological Chemistry* (2003).

Lethaby, Anne, Jane Marjoribanks, Fredi Kronenberg, Helen Roberts, John Eden, and Julie Brown. "Phytoestrogens for menopausal vasomotor symptoms." *Cochrane Database of Systematic Reviews* 12 (2013).

Lippman, Scott M., Eric A. Klein, Phyllis J. Goodman, M. Scott Lucia, Ian M. Thompson, Leslie G. Ford, Howard L. Parnes, Lori M. Minasian, J. Michael Gaziano, Jo Ann Hartline, J. Kellogg Parsons, James D. Bearden, E. David Crawford, Gary E. Goodman, Jaime Claudio, Eric Winquist, Elise D. Cook, Daniel D. Karp, Philip Walther, Michael M. Lieber, Alan R. Kristal, Amy K. Darke, Kathryn B. Arnold, Patricia A. Ganz, Regina M. Santella, Demetrius Albanes, Philip R. Taylor, Jeffrey L. Probstfield, T. J. Jagpal, John J. Crowley, Frank L. Meyskens, Laurence H. Baker, and Charles A. Coltman. "Effect of selenium and vitamin E on risk of prostate cancer and other cancers: the Selenium and Vitamin E Cancer Prevention Trial (SELECT)." *Jama* 301, no. 1 (2009): 39-51.

Lisa Simonson. "Is Goat Meat Healthy," accessed on October 6, 2017. https://www.livestrong.com/article/367559-is-goat-meat-healthy/.

Lunn, J., and H. E. Theobald. "The health effects of dietary unsaturated fatty acids." *Nutrition Bulletin* 31, no. 3 (2006): 178-224.

Luqmani, Y. A. "Mechanisms of drug resistance in cancer chemotherapy." *Medical Principles and Practice* 14, no. Suppl. 1 (2005): 35-48.

MacLennan, Mira B., Shannon E. Clarke, Kate Perez, Geoffrey A. Wood, William J. Muller, Jing X. Kang, and David WL Ma. "Mammary tumor development is directly inhibited by lifelong n-3 polyunsaturated fatty acids." *The Journal of Nutritional Biochemistry* 24, no. 1 (2013): 388-395.

McIntosh, Graeme H. "Cereal foods, fibres and the prevention of cancers." *Australian Journal of Nutrition and Dietetics* 58, no. 4 (2001): S35-S35.

Mehta, Reema D., and Andrew J. Roth. "Psychiatric considerations in the oncology setting." *CA: A Cancer Journal for Clinicians* 65, no. 4 (2015): 299-314.

Mukhtar, Hasan, and Nihal Ahmad. "Tea polyphenols: prevention of cancer and optimizing health." *The American Journal of Clinical Nutrition* 71, no. 6 (2000): 1698S-1702S.

Murillo, Genoveva, and Rajendra G. Mehta. "Cruciferous vegetables and cancer prevention." *Nutrition and Cancer* 41, no. 1-2 (2001): 17-28.

National Cancer Institute, "Cruciferous Vegetables and Cancer Prevention.", accessed on August 13, 2016. https://www.cancer.gov/about-cancer/causes-prevention/risk/diet/cruciferous-vegetables-fact-sheet.

NHLBI Obesity Education Initiative Expert Panel on the Identification, Evaluation, and Treatment of Obesity in Adults (US). *Clinical Guidelines on the Identification, Evaluation, and Treatment of Overweight and Obesity in Adults: The Evidence Report*. Bethesda (MD): National Heart, Lung, and Blood Institute; 1998 Sep. Available at: https://www.ncbi.nlm.nih.gov/books/NBK2003/

Nelson, David E., Dwayne W. Jarman, Jürgen Rehm, Thomas K. Greenfield, Grégoire Rey, William C. Kerr, Paige Miller, Kevin D. Shield, Yu Ye, and Timothy S. Naimi. "Alcohol-attributable Cancer Deaths and Years of Potential Life Lost in the United States." *American Journal of Public Health* 103, no. 4 (2013): 641-648.

Nichols, Kim E., David Malkin, Judy E. Garber, Joseph F. Fraumeni, and Frederick P. Li. "Germ-line p53 mutations predispose to a wide spectrum of early-onset cancers." *Cancer Epidemiology and Prevention Biomarkers* 10, no. 2 (2001): 83-87.

Nieman, David C., Nicholas D. Gillitt, Amy M. Knab, R. Andrew Shanely, Kirk L. Pappan, Fuxia Jin, and Mary Ann Lila. "Influence of a polyphenol-enriched protein powder on exercise-induced inflammation and oxidative stress in athletes: a randomized trial using a metabolomics approach." *PLoS One* 8, no. 8 (2013): e72215.

Nussbaum, Martha, and Amartya Sen, eds. *The Quality of Life*. Oxford: Oxford University Press, 1993.

Ogden, Cynthia L., Margaret D. Carroll, Cheryl D. Fryar, and Katherine M. Flegal. *Prevalence of obesity among adults and youth: United States, 2011-2014*. Washington, DC: US Department of Health and Human Services, Centers for Disease Control and Prevention, National Center for Health Statistics, 2015.

Parker, C., S. Nilsson, Daniel Heinrich, Svein I. Helle, J. M. O'Sullivan, Sophie D. Fosså, Aleš Chodacki, John Logue, Peter Hoskin, David Bottomley, Nicholas D. James, Isabel Syndikus, Robert Coleman, Mihalj Seke, Anders Widmark, Lars Franzén, Dag Clement Johannessen, Charles Gillies O'Bryan-Tear, Karin Staudacher, Øyvind S. Bruland, Arne Solberg, Paweł Wiechno, Jan Kliment, Steffen Wedel, Sibylle Boehmer, Marcos Dall'Oglio, Nicholas J. Vogelzang, Jose GarciaVargas, and Oliver Sartor. "Alpha emitter radium-223 and survival in metastatic prostate cancer." *New England Journal of Medicine* 369, no. 3 (2013): 213-223.

Per, Hüseyin, Selim Kurtoğlu, Fatih Yağmur, Hakan Gümüş, Sefer Kumandaş, and M. Hakan Poyrazoğlu. "Calcium carbide poisoning via food in childhood." *The Journal of Emergency Medicine* 32, no. 2 (2007): 179-180.

Pirl, William F. "Evidence report on the occurrence, assessment, and treatment of depression in cancer patients." *JNCI Monographs* 2004, no. 32 (2004): 32-39.

Prakash, Usha N.S. and Krishnapura Srinivasan. "Gastrointestinal protective effect of dietary spices during ethanol-induced oxidant stress in experimental rats." *Applied Physiology, Nutrition, and Metabolism* 35, no. 2 (2010): 134-141.

Praud, Delphine, Matteo Rota, Jürgen Rehm, Kevin Shield, Witold Zatoski, Mia Hashibe, Carlo La Vecchia, and Paolo Boffetta. "Cancer incidence and mortality attributable to alcohol consumption." *International Journal of Cancer* 138, no. 6 (2016): 1380-1387.

Nitin Rao, Araga Ramesha Rao, Laxmi Narayna Jannu, and Syed Perwez Hussain. "Chemoprevention of 7, 12-Dimethylbenz [a] anthracene-induced Mammary Carcinogenesis in Rat by the Combined Actions of Selenium, Magnesium, Ascorbic Acid and Retinyl Acetate." *Japanese Journal of Cancer Research* 81, no. 12 (1990): 1239-1246.

Reddy, M. N., N. Rajashekhar Reddy, and K. Jamil. "Spicy anti-cancer spices: A review." *International Journal of Pharmacy and Pharmaceutical Sciences* 7, no. 11 (2015): 1-6.

Renehan, Andrew G., Jan Frystyk, and Allan Flyvbjerg. "Obesity and cancer risk: the role of the insulin–IGF axis." *Trends in Endocrinology & Metabolism* 17, no. 8 (2006): 328-336.

Renwick, Andrew G. "The intake of intense sweeteners–an update review." *Food Additives and Contaminants* 23, no. 4 (2006): 327-338.

Riley, Todd, Eduardo Sontag, Patricia Chen, and Arnold Levine. "Transcriptional control of human p53-regulated genes." *Nature Reviews Molecular Cell Biology* 9, no. 5 (2008): 402.

Roberts, Darren L., Caroline Dive, and Andrew G. Renehan. "Biological mechanisms linking obesity and cancer risk: new perspectives." *Annual Review of Medicine* 61 (2010): 301-316.

Robison, Alice K., David A. Sirbasku, and George M. Stancel. "DDT supports the growth of an estrogen-responsive tumor: mammary tumor growth; pesticides." *Toxicology Letters* 27, no. 1-3 (1985): 109-113.

Rock, Cheryl L., Colleen Doyle, Wendy Demark-Wahnefried, Jeffrey Meyerhardt, Kerry S. Courneya, Anna L. Schwartz, Elisa V. Bandera Kathryn K. Hamilton, Barbara Grant, Marji McCullough, Tim Byers and Ted Gansler. "Nutrition and physical activity guidelines for cancer survivors." *CA: A Cancer Journal For Clinicians* 62, no. 4 (2012): 242-274.

Rodin, Gary, Nancy Lloyd, Mark Katz, Esther Green, Jean A. Mackay, Rebecca KS Wong, and Supportive Care Guidelines Group of Cancer Care Ontario Program in Evidence-Based Care. "The treatment of depression in cancer patients: a systematic review." *Supportive Care in Cancer* 15, no. 2 (2007): 123-136.

Ryter, Stefan W., Hong Pyo Kim, Alexander Hoetzel, Jeong W. Park, Kiichi Nakahira, Xue Wang, and Augustine MK Choi. "Mechanisms of cell death in oxidative stress." *Antioxidants & Redox Signaling* 9, no. 1 (2007): 49-89.

Safdie, Fernando M., Tanya Dorff, David Quinn, Luigi Fontana, Min Wei, Changhan Lee, Pinchas Cohen, and Valter D. Longo. "Fasting and cancer treatment in humans: A case series report." *Aging (Albany NY)* 1, no. 12 (2009): 988.

Scadden, David T. "AIDS-related malignancies." *Annual Review of Medicine* 54, no. 1 (2003): 285-303.

Schloerb, Paul R. "Immune-enhancing diets: products, components, and their rationales." *Journal of Parenteral and Enteral Nutrition* 25, no. 2 (2001): S3-S7.

Seitz, Helmut K., and Felix Stickel. "Molecular mechanisms of alcohol-mediated carcinogenesis." *Nature Reviews Cancer* 7, no. 8 (2007): 599.

Séralini, Gilles-Eric, Dominique Cellier, and Joël Spiroux de Vendomois. "New analysis of a rat feeding study with a genetically modified maize reveals signs of hepatorenal toxicity." *Archives of Environmental Contamination and Toxicology* 52, no. 4 (2007): 596-602.

Shekhar, P. V. M., J. Werdell, and V. S. Basrur. "Environmental estrogen stimulation of growth and estrogen receptor function in preneoplastic and cancerous human breast cell lines." *Journal of the National Cancer Institute* 89, no. 23 (1997): 1774-1782.

Siddiqui, Md Wasim, and R. S. Dhua. "Eating artificially ripened fruits is harmful." *Current Science* (2010): 1664-1668.

Silvestri, Gerard A., Sommer Knittig, James S. Zoller, and Paul J. Nietert. "Importance of faith on medical decisions regarding cancer care." *Journal of Clinical Oncology* 21, no. 7 (2003): 1379-1382.

Simopoulos, Artemis P. "The importance of the omega-6/omega-3 fatty acid ratio in cardiovascular disease and other chronic diseases." *Experimental Biology and Medicine* 233, no. 6 (2008): 674-688.

Singhi, P. D. "Newer antiepileptic drugs and non-surgical approaches in epilepsy." *Indian Journal of Pediatrics* 67, no. 1 Suppl (2000): S92-8.

Soffritti, Morando, Fiorella Belpoggi, Davide Degli Esposti, Luca Lambertini, Eva Tibaldi, and Anna Rigano. "First experimental demonstration of the multipotential carcinogenic effects of aspartame administered in the feed to Sprague-Dawley rats." *Environmental Health Perspectives* 114, no. 3 (2005): 379-385.

Sood, Amit, and Timothy J. Moynihan. "Cancer-related fatigue: an update." *Current Oncology Reports* 7, no. 4 (2005): 277-282.

Southwick, Steven M., Meena Vythilingam, and Dennis S. Charney. "The psychobiology of depression and resilience to stress: implications for prevention and treatment." *Annual Review of Clinical Psychoogy* 1 (2005): 255-291.

Stevenson, Mario. "HIV-1 pathogenesis." *Nature Medicine* 9, no. 7 (2003): 853.

Tachino, Nicholas, Dexin Guo, Wan Mohaiza Dashwood, Shane Yamane, Randy Larsen, and Roderick Dashwood. "Mechanisms of the in vitro antimutagenic action of chlorophyllin against benzo [a] pyrene: studies of enzyme inhibition, molecular complex formation and degradation of the ultimate carcinogen." *Mutation Research/ Fundamental and Molecular Mechanisms of Mutagenesis* 308, no. 2 (1994): 191-203.

Temel, Jennifer S., Joseph A. Greer, Alona Muzikansky, Emily R. Gallagher, Sonal Admane, Vicki A. Jackson, Constance M. Dahlin, Craig D. Blinderman, Juliet Jacobsen, William F. Pirl, J. Andrew Billings, and Thomas J. Lynch. "Early palliative care for patients with metastatic non–small-cell lung cancer." *New England Journal of Medicine* 363, no. 8 (2010): 733-742.

Tordoff, Michael G., and Annette M. Alleva. "Effect of drinking soda sweetened with aspartame or high-fructose corn syrup on food intake and body weight." *The American Journal of Clinical Nutrition* 51, no. 6 (1990): 963-969.

Devita, Vincent T., Theodore S. Lawrence and Steven A. Rosenberg eds. *Cancer: Principles & Practice of Oncology*. Philadelphia: Lippincott William & Wilkins, 2011.

Trock, Bruce J., Leena Hilakivi-Clarke, and Robert Clarke. "Meta-analysis of soy intake and breast cancer risk." *Journal of the National Cancer Institute* 98, no. 7 (2006): 459-471.

Valko, Marian, Dieter Leibfritz, Jan Moncol, Mark TD Cronin, Milan Mazur, and Joshua Telser. "Free radicals and antioxidants in normal physiological functions and human disease." *The international journal of biochemistry & cell biology* 39, no. 1 (2007): 44-84.

van Frankenhuyzen, Kees. "The challenge of Bacillus thuringiensis." In *Bacillus Thuringiensis, An Environmental Biopesticide: Theory and Practice.* Hoboken: John Wiley & Sons, 1993.

Vasanthi, R. Hannah, and R. P. Parameswari. "Indian spices for healthy heart-an overview." *Current Cardiology Reviews* 6, no. 4 (2010): 274-279.

Watson, Cheryl S., Yow-Jiun Jeng, and Jutatip Guptarak. "Endocrine disruption via estrogen receptors that participate in nongenomic signaling pathways." *The Journal of Steroid Biochemistry and Molecular Biology* 127, no. 1-2 (2011): 44-50.

Wei, Chia-Lin, Qiang Wu, Vinsensius B. Vega, Kuo Ping Chiu, Patrick Ng, Tao Zhang, Atif Shahab, How Choong Yong, Yu Tao Fu, Zhiping Weng, Jian Jun Liu, Xiao Dong Zhao, Joon-Lin Chew, Yen Ling Lee, Vladimir A. Kuznetsov, Wing-Kin Sung, Lance D. Miller, Bing Lim, Edison T. Liu, Qiang Yu, Huck-Hui Ng, and Yijun Ruan. "A global map of p53 transcription-factor binding sites in the human genome." *Cell* 124, no. 1 (2006): 207-219.

Wilken, Reason, Mysore S. Veena, Marilene B. Wang, and Eri S. Srivatsan. "Curcumin: A review of anti-cancer properties and therapeutic activity in head and neck squamous cell carcinoma." *Molecular Cancer* 10, no. 1 (2011): 12.

Wolff, Antonio C., M. Elizabeth H. Hammond, David G. Hicks, Mitch Dowsett, Lisa M. McShane, Kimberly H. Allison, Donald C. Allred, John M.S. Bartlett, Michael Bilous, Patrick Fitzgibbons, Wedad Hanna, Robert B. Jenkins, Pamela B. Mangu, Soonmyung Paik, Edith A. Perez, Michael F. Press, Patricia A. Spears, Gail H. Vance, Giuseppe Viale, and Daniel F. Hayes. "Recommendations for human epidermal growth factor receptor 2 testing in breast cancer: American Society of Clinical Oncology/College of American Pathologists clinical practice guideline update." *Archives of Pathology and Laboratory Medicine* 138, no. 2 (2013): 241-256.

Wu, A. H., M. C. Yu, C. C. Tseng, and M. C. Pike. "Epidemiology of soy exposures and breast cancer risk." *British Journal of Cancer* 98, no. 1 (2008): 9.

Yarbro, Connie Henke, Debra Wujcik, and Barbara Holmes Gobel. *Cancer Symptom Management*. Boston: Jones & Bartlett Learning, 2013.

Yokoyama, Akira, and Tai Omori. "Genetic polymorphisms of alcohol and aldehyde dehydrogenases and risk for esophageal and head and neck cancers." *Japanese Journal of Clinical Oncology* 33, no. 3 (2003): 111-121.

Zahreddine, Hiba, and Katherine Borden. "Mechanisms and insights into drug resistance in cancer." *Frontiers in Pharmacology* 4 (2013): 28.

Glossary

ADT: Androgen deprivation therapy.

Anaerobe: An organism that does not require oxygen for it growth. Cancer cells are anaerobic.

Anions: Atoms that have gained an electron and have a negative charge.

Angiogenesis: New blood vessel formation.

Apoptosis: A process of programmed cell death.

Carcinogen: Cancer-causing substance.

Carotenoids: Plant pigments responsible for the colour of fruits and vegetables, which act as antioxidants and can get converted into Vitamin A.

CD-4: Lymphocytes that play a major role in protecting the body against infections.

Cachexia: A wasting syndrome with loss of weight, muscle atrophy, fatigue and significant loss of appetite in a cancer patient, or any patient with a long-standing chronic debilitating disease.

CLL: Chronic lymphocytic leukaemia.

Cytotoxic agent: The quality of being toxic to the cells, like chemotherapeutic drugs.

Cox 2 enzyme: A pro-inflammatory substance that is harmful to the nuclear membrane.

DNA: Deoxyribonucleic acid is a molecule that carries genetic instructions used in growth, development and functioning of all multi-cellular organisms.

Epigenetic factor: Factors that interact with genetic material but do not change the DNA sequence, acting as chemical tags that indicate when the gene should turn 'on'.

FISH: Fluorescence in-situ hybridization.

Flavonoids: Antioxidants in plant-based foods that prevent cell damage.

Gleeson score: A system of grading prostate cancer based on microscope appearance.

GM: Genetically modified crops. Their DNA is modified by genetic engineering techniques.

HER 2: Human epithelial growth factor receptor 2.

HIV-AIDS: Acquired immune deficiency syndrome caused by infection of the human immunodeficiency virus.

Hyperinsulinemia: Excessive levels of insulin relative to the levels of glucose circulating in the blood.

Hyperbaric oxygen: Medical treatment which enhances the body's natural healing process by inhalation of 100 per cent oxygen in a total body chamber.

Mitochondria: Structures within the cells that store and generate most of the cells' energy as chemical energy—the power house of the cell.

MSG: Monosodium glutamate; a non-essential amino acid used as a flavouring agent in junk food.

Mutation: Alteration in the chemical structure of the DNA.

Neurotransmitters: Chemical messengers that transmit signals across a chemical synapse or from one neuron to another.

NK cells: Cytotoxic lymphocytes critical to the innate immune system and the first defence against cancer cells.

Omega-3: Essential fatty acid for normal metabolism.

Oxidative stress: The structural cellular damage that occurs due to chemical reactions with chemical species containing oxygen-like peroxide or super-oxides generated within the cell.

p53: The gene that codes for a protein which regulates the cell cycle and therefore functions as a tumour suppressor.

Phagocytic cells: White blood cells that protect the body by ingesting harmful foreign particles, bacteria and dead cells.

Phytoestrogens: Plant-derived oestrogens.

Polyphenols: Natural organic chemicals characterized by the presence of large multiple phenol structural units; found in tea.

Phytonutrients: Plant-derived nutrients.

PSA: Prostate-specific antigen.

Selenium: A trace element that is naturally present in many foods and is nutritionally essential for humans in reproduction, thyroid hormone metabolism, DNA synthesis and provides protection from oxidative stress.

Telomere: A region of repetitive nucleotide sequence at each end of a chromosome which protects the ends of the chromosome from deteriorating and shortening with age.

Xenoestrogens: A hormone that imitates oestrogen and can be either synthetic or a natural chemical compound.